When Glad Becomes Sad

When Glad Becomes Sad

Personal Accounts From People Living With Depression

KAREN Z. HENDIN

iUniverse, Inc.

New York   Bloomington

When Glad Becomes Sad
Personal Accounts From People Living With Depression

iUniverse books may be ordered through booksellers or by contacting:

iUniverse
1663 Liberty Drive
Bloomington, IN 47403
www.iuniverse.com
1-800-Authors (1-800-288-4677)

ISBN: 978-0-595-52901-8 (pbk)
ISBN: 978-0-595-51990-3 (cloth)
ISBN: 978-0-595-62951-0 (ebk)

Printed in the United States of America

iUniverse rev. date: 1/19/2009

Disclaimer

When Glad Becomes Sad is presented as a collection of stories of personal experiences. This book does not endorse or guarantee the efficacy of any action, practice, or medication mentioned herein. The individual accounts are not intended to replace or supersede medical consultation or treatment.

In loving memory of my mother

Contents

Preface

The intent of this book is to provide a source of support for people who experience depression or anxiety disorders, as well as their families and friends. In my own struggles with depression, it was difficult to find a book of this nature that was not complicated by the use of medical terms beyond a layman's comprehension.

Aside from the professional help I am fortunate to have in my life, I have spent hours researching the internet, reading books and speaking with people in search of the support I feel that I require.

I have a Bachelor of Arts degree with a major in Psychology from the University of Manitoba. My husband and I ran a small business for approximately twenty-five years. It was during this time that I pursued a Certificate in Business Administration with a major in Accounting from Red River College.

I then enrolled in the Applied Counseling Skills Program at Red River College. I completed a practicum in an emergency department of a Winnipeg hospital assessing lethality.

Once out in the field, I gained extensive knowledge in working both with mentally challenged adults and children. I have managed a group home, and have had experience working in classrooms, daycares and personal care homes.

I have volunteered at several schools in Winnipeg as well as with social service organizations. My volunteer experience has also included visiting palliative care patients and facilitating bereavement support groups.

Professionally, I have conducted workshops in an extended education program in a Winnipeg school division. The topics included Stress Management, Time Management, Meditation, Humor, and Exceptional Customer Service.

I have also spoken to networking groups and seniors' organizations. I have spoken at conferences as well, one of the most notable having been The Manitoba Hospice and Palliative Care Conference in 2004.

I am currently conducting personal and professional development workshops in a private practice. I regularly attend seminars and conferences that will enhance my abilities as a consultant.

I am also attending courses at University of Manitoba working towards a Certificate in Teaching English as an Additional Language. For the past eight years, I have volunteered in this field in a program for adults in a Winnipeg school division.

I have completed the Leadership Training Program at the YMCA-YWCA in Winnipeg. This certification enables me to volunteer at the YMCA-YWCA teaching Aquafit classes.

I was also recently recognized as a '*Hero*' at an event held by the Canadian Mental Health Association in Winnipeg. I am truly honored that Marleen at the YMCA-YWCA West Portage had nominated me.

When Glad Becomes Sad is my first self-published book. It has been an incredible learning experience. Friends are asking me if I intend to write another book. Anything is possible.

Acknowledgements

A heartfelt thank you to all of the brave people who submitted their stories outlining their experiences while struggling with depression. Your contributions have made this book possible.

David, Lise, Cheyenna, and Rita; you are the greatest friends and have all become an important part of my extended family.

Av, we were not only cousins but we shared a very close friendship throughout our lives which I will always treasure in my heart. I hope you have found peace now.

I would also like to acknowledge the members of The Manitoba Christian Writing Association. I have met an incredible group of women and men with a wealth of information to share.

Special thanks to Dr. B.J. Armstrong; without your support and encouragement over the years, I highly doubt that I'd be here today, with this book completed and another goal achieved. Your assistance in editing the medical terminology and medication sections is also greatly appreciated.

Koal, there are no words to express just how much your unconditional love and companionship has meant to me over the years. I only wish you could have lived forever.

K-Team; you are the loves of my life! I revel in your accomplishments and now it's time for you to share in mine.

Introduction

I have lived with a major or clinical depression that was first diagnosed twelve years ago. The initial purpose of this book was to tell my story. My friends convinced me that there are many people out there who would be anxious to share their experiences. Judging by the number of stories I have received, depression is running rampant in our society today. People feel the need to talk, but they also seek anonymity.

Along with my return address, I distributed guidelines in envelopes randomly to members of the community. The original guidelines were quite wordy. I then distributed additional envelopes that contained the revised guidelines as follows:

I am currently writing a book dealing with depression. I am not a psychiatrist or a psychologist. I am just like you. I live with depression every day of my life. This book is intended for you and me and is not another clinical study by a professional. You will not need a medical dictionary by your side. Our contributions are the stories you will find in this book.

I hope that you will feel comfortable sharing your experiences. Be assured that anyone who contributes will remain strictly anonymous. I have not numbered the envelopes and I ask that you do not write your name on your papers or on the envelope.

Feel free to write as much or as little as you would like to. You may wish to write about your own experience with depression. You may have cared for or lived with someone suffering from depression. You may have known someone who has attempted or who has succeeded in committing suicide.

Or you may have had absolutely no experience with depression.

Depression often causes marriages to break up, families to become estranged, drastic changes in behavior, and sometimes results in addictions as well. Unfortunately too many people are unaware of what depression is and do not understand the experiences that they are having.

Each of us has a unique story to tell. Upon reading the completed book your self-esteem and morale are sure to rise when you see that others have had similar experiences and have survived. They may have valuable information to pass on. You may have been diagnosed as having a specific type of depression. If you have never sought professional help in the past, this book may encourage you to do so. And if you are living with someone who suffers from depression, I hope that this book will help you to better understand this condition.

Imagine that you are sharing your experience with a friend. View this as an exercise in expressing your true feelings regarding depression. Remember, you will remain anonymous.

I ask that you write honestly and sincerely. Please include appropriate details in your story such as your age, marital status, and whether you live in an urban or rural area.

Please include details such as if you have ever sought professional help, how you felt prior to receiving help, how you felt when the professional confirmed a diagnosis, your feelings regarding medication(s), if you are still on medication and how you feel now as compared with how you felt prior.

How as all this impacted on family and other social relationships? Has this affected you at work? Has this affected any volunteer work you do? Has your sex life been affected? Have you been able to cope with house cleaning and financial management? Has this experience had an effect on your self-image? How is your self-esteem and morale? Has your weight fluctuated? Has your general appearance changed? Have you ever attended a support group or psychotherapy sessions?

Are you completely familiar with any medications you are currently on (or have been on in the past)? Have you noticed any physical side effects? Has your sleep been affected? How is your energy level? Have you experienced headaches, digestive problems, dry-mouth, sweating, or anxiety?

The above may cover a period of days, weeks, months, or years. They may change at any point in time and may change several times, especially when there is a change in medication.

How would you describe your state of health and/or mind now? How has (have) your medications affected your health and/or mind set?

The above guidelines are to offer direction and to remind you of the finer points of your story. There is no wrong way to write your contribution. You are a unique individual.

Thank you so much for agreeing to share your experiences with others. This type of book is one that we will all cherish as we will identify with the emotions and physical symptoms of each other. Good luck in your writing! I have every confidence that our effort will be a success.

Karen

In editing the stories in this book, only spelling has been corrected. The content and grammar have not been changed in any way. To do so would change the tone and the authenticity of each submission.

I have also included some statistics regarding mental health issues. These may be found at the back of the book following the stories.

Of great importance is the fact that when you read this book, you will not require a medical dictionary or a pharmaceutical directory. With the help of Dr. B. J. Armstrong, I have compiled a list of common medical terminology as well as medications used today. These may be found at the end of the book following the statistics. Some of these terms and drug names may be mentioned in stories that people have submitted, or they may be familiar to you in your own experiences with depression.

I have also included a resource list at the end of the book. These are a sampling only of the many valuable resources available. There are hundreds of sites on the internet. The ones listed in my book are sites that I have found useful in both my personal and professional life.

I have organized the book in terms of the many different types of depression and anxiety disorders. You will note that there is some overlap in some instances. It is my sincere hope that when reading the stories of others who live with depression, their experiences will be a source of support and encouragement for you.

Author's Story

It's happening again. It hurts too much to breathe. My head feels heavy and my body feels numb. I am devoid of energy and couldn't care less about anyone or anything in my life. I've come very close to dying four times in the last three years. It's something I live with everyday. It's impossible to dismiss it from my mind. But somehow I manage, day by day, to slowly let the gloominess pass. This is how depression has affected me.

There is a big difference between wanting to die and attempting suicide, and wanting to live only to have someone else try to end your life. Unfortunately I have experienced both, and they have had a great impact on my life.

Depression is often referred to as a silent killer. Years ago people who exhibited signs of mental disorders were often locked up in institutions as they were considered dangerous and violent. They were seen as a menace to society, and it was assumed that they were harmful to not only themselves but to others as well. These people were often pitied and misunderstood. The common belief was that once people were institutionalized, there was no hope for them and they certainly had no rightful place in society. Instead, they were best off in strait jackets and treated with electric shock. Thankfully these barbaric practices are no longer as common. Today there are medications available that help to keep the chemicals in our brains in balance.

Some people experience depression that lasts a short time. I have not been as fortunate. I struggle with a clinical or major depression every single day of my life. In all probability I will require daily medication for the rest of my life. It is a challenge in itself to find the right medication, as adjustments are required periodically. These drugs also have some unpleasant side effects. But the benefits derived are well worth the effort.

My experience with depression began several years ago when my life became complicated and turbulent. My mother died very unexpectedly after having knee replacement surgery. Instead of being discharged from the hospital on my birthday, she was moved to a medical intensive care unit. This began a four week long roller coaster ride of emotions which eventually culminated in her death. I felt betrayed by the medical professionals. Something had gone very wrong after the surgery, and they were unable to determine what it was in time to save her life.

Shortly after my mother's death, family problems arose when it was time to settle the estate. It was obvious that my mother had been greatly influenced and manipulated by a needy family member. Rectifying this situation would have involved legal recourse on my part. Aside from the obvious outrageous legal fees, I felt that emotionally I could not deal with another ugly situation at this time. I declined all offers of legal assistance from many lawyers. There is no revenge that will ever compensate for the hurt and betrayal that I felt.

There were a lot of other changes that occurred in my life. My husband and I sold our business. We sold the building that the business had occupied. Ken was unemployed for a while and I went back to school. Ken changed careers and I began a new career once I graduated. We then moved from Tuxedo to a community just outside of the city.

In the spring of 2005, Ken and I became empty-nesters. It was quite an adjustment for both of us. Unfortunately, all it did was exacerbate the stormy relationship we had experienced for quite some time now. To say that I was unhappy was an understatement. We had tried going for counseling, but it seemed like an exercise in futility.

By the first week in June, I was feeling terribly overwhelmed and very down. It was time to say good-bye and get off the merry-go-round. I'd had enough fun. I had a very busy week. I met Cheyenna for our annual birthday dinner. I spent a day with Lise. I sat with Rita at an auction. I visited David at school. And I spent time with my children. On Friday Ken and I had an appointment together with our psychiatrist. I totally alienated Ken to the point where he walked out of the session. My work was done.

I spent most of the weekend sleeping. On Sunday night I sent an email to my husband. I knew he wouldn't be checking his email until he got to work Monday morning. I took double the medication I usually take at bedtime. I got up and took my dog out for a walk. I then came in, climbed into bed, and swallowed more Lorazepam and Temazepam. I remember waking up a few times; realizing I was still alive, and wondering how many more pills I had to take. I just took a few more every time I woke up. My memory cuts out here. My husband says he came home and he called my doctor. A couple of days later I remember deciding to cut out all medication, and I wound up in a hospital emergency ward in the middle of the night.

Two months later I was diagnosed as having osteoarthritis in my knees. The surgery that I must look forward to is the one that my mother died from. Having no faith in our healthcare system at this point, I went to the Mayo Clinic rather than wait several months to see a specialist in Winnipeg. I followed their advice and within two weeks I was walking again. Apparently the leg brace (provided to me by Manitoba Health) was wreaking havoc on my good knee, my hips and my back. The physio I had been doing was also inappropriate.

When I returned from the Mayo Clinic, I joined the West Branch of the YMCA-YWCA in Winnipeg. I tentatively attempted two shallow aquafit classes per week. As I felt better, I attended more classes. It's been over two years now, and I have graduated to deep water classes and I do not use a flotation device anymore. Never in my wildest dreams did I ever think that I would be doing deep water aquafit classes six times a week.

In the summer of 2007 I had another experience with betrayal when a doctor made a grave error in prescribing medication. One day I passed out in the driveway and banged my head on a concrete step. I was experiencing hypokalemia due to an overdose of potassium. I was totally shocked at the reaction from my doctor. The last thing I needed to hear was insinuations that I was the one who had taken the wrong dose. Dying was not on my agenda at that time. Here I was, determined to get my life back on track, when it could just as easily have been snuffed out by someone else's error.

It is important to understand that with the aid of medication I can lead a productive life. I no longer procrastinate and psyche myself up when I need to go out. The tranquilizers have become a memory. I realize how fortunate I am to have a caring and compassionate psychiatrist in my life, and I value greatly the support from my family and friends as well.

Following are some suggestions that have helped me in dealing with depression. These ideas are not meant to take the place of professional help or medications. While there is no guarantee that they will be helpful for everyone, I do encourage that you try some of them.

I strongly feel that journaling is a valuable tool when dealing with depression. It may be more comfortable to write than to express these feelings aloud. Written contemplation of events often assists in the recognition of triggers as well.

This past winter, I purchased a desk lamp that I feel benefits not only people who suffer from Seasonal Affective Disorder, but any type of depression. The fluorescent bulbs give off a light that is comparable to natural daylight. This lamp has also helped on the gloomier days this past spring and summer. These lamps are readily available at several stores locally or may be ordered on-line. Another plus is that they are relatively inexpensive. I prefer the desk model as I can move it from room to room. Whether I'm at the computer or reading in bed, this lamp has been most effective. I also have the same type of lighting in the fluorescent fixture in my kitchen.

Exercising on a regular basis is highly recommended. I attend aquafit and/or fitness classes on a daily basis. I prefer to be in the pool early in the morning and I find it a great way to start my day. Both my physical and mental health have improved with this routine. My energy level has increased as has my self-esteem.

I also carefully watch the amount of caffeine I have everyday. I definitely advise avoiding caffeine at night, especially if sleeping is affected by depression. Alcohol and recreational usage of drugs are other areas to be monitored, as they can alter the effectiveness of anti-depressants and anti-anxiety medications.

I make a point of finding time for myself. I have practiced meditation for years and have shared my knowledge with others. Relaxation is a wonderful tool in combating the stress that may cause or complicate a depression disorder.

I can't emphasize enough the importance of setting realistic goals. Satisfaction and a feeling of accomplishment are far better than frustration and disappointment. When a goal is achieved, I congratulate myself, acknowledging that I have just passed another milestone in life.

By working together with a competent professional, I have come to realize the importance of taking prescription medication as instructed. When the sad times do happen, my coping skills that have developed during my treatment now enable me to deal with these situations in a healthier manner. One of the most significant realizations has been that when I do need to ask for help, I no longer view it as a sign of weakness. Although people have often come to rely on me, it is only recently that I have learned to say to others *"I need to talk"*.

We are all familiar with the expression *"Honesty is the best policy"*. Be honest with yourself about your feelings. Be honest with your therapist about what is happening in your life. Honesty is an important part of the hard work needed in dealing with depression.

I sincerely hope that in the future, additional research will enable a diagnosis to be reached more accurately and quickly, so that immediate and appropriate treatment can be made available to those of us who suffer from depression. In the meantime, I take comfort in knowing that there are drugs that will in most cases ensure a reasonable quality of life. Compare this with people who have been diagnosed with aggressive forms of cancer. There are no pills that will improve their health.

I hope you will derive the same comfort and peace when reading this book as I did when editing and writing it. I like to think that this is a readily available support system in book form. By identifying with the experiences of others I realize that I am not alone.

Contributor's Stories Part 1: Major Depression

I had absolutely no idea what depression was until my husband was diagnosed with it five years ago. My husband was hospitalized in order to receive the proper treatment and supervision that he required. He was given anti-depressants and tranquilizers.

My children were quite young and terrified of their father. They insisted on barricading the front door with furniture in case he escaped from the hospital. I was extremely worried about my children. As if this wasn't enough to contend with, I had the most non-supportive extended family members imaginable.

For several months I had to work, care for my children and pretend that life was normal. I had very little contact with my husband at that time. My imagination ran wild and I saw myself as a single parent at age forty with two teenagers.

My husband was seeing a psychiatrist regularly. He phoned me one day and told me that he was being discharged and intended to move in with his brother. He also informed me that his doctor would like me to attend his next session. My first reaction was anger. I wasn't the one who was depressed. I wasn't the one who abandoned the family. But I was curious, so I agreed to meet him at the doctor's office. His psychiatrist urged me to attend as many sessions as I could so that I would understand what my husband was experiencing.

It was really hard work adjusting to the changes in my husband's behavior. When he did return home, the children were afraid of him and tried to stay away from him. They both had too many memories of his outbursts and moods. To this day they wish that I had divorced him.

I often wonder what life would have been like had we divorced at that time. Obviously my scars haven't healed yet either.

*****

D	Devastated
E	Everyday
P	Pressured
R	Reclusive
E	Emptiness
S	Sad
S	Suicide
I	I'm a failure
O	Ornery
N	No Energy

*****

Right now I feel sad. I don't know why. I got up this morning and had a leisurely cup of coffee while reading the newspaper. I soaked in a tub full of fragrant bubbles. I decided to treat myself to a manicure and a pedicure at a spa nearby. I came home and took a nice long nap. My children are at their uncle's farm for the weekend. My husband is away on another business trip for a week. I live a pampered and privileged life. Our home is as big as a palace. I drive a fancy car. I have more clothes and shoes than some women have in a lifetime. Other women envy me all the luxuries that I enjoy.

I've always been a quiet person. I've always kept my thoughts to myself. Sometimes I feel like a robot that goes through life without any real feelings about anything. It seems like everything is always decided for me and that plans always work out perfectly. Please don't misunderstand me. I have a wonderful and generous husband who will probably bring me back another fabulous piece of jewelry when he returns from his business trip. I love my twin girls to pieces, but they are at that age where they are just experimenting with their newfound lives as teenagers. I have always encouraged them to be creative and to reach for the stars. As a result, one of them is an all-star athlete who is talented in every sport imaginable. We have a basketball net in our driveway and a tennis court in the backyard. The girls both have horses that they board at their uncle's farm. My other daughter is very musically talented. She plays the flute, the piccolo and the harp. She is constantly performing and she has her very own harp in a music room that was built for her in the basement.

On the surface my life appears to be an ideal one. I lack for nothing. And this is why I feel so confused that I cry and feel sad all the time.

I tried going to a therapist once. She was a lovely woman who had some very inspiring ideas to help bring me out of my shell. But somehow I just never got around to joining an art club and learning to paint, or trying my hand at ceramics or pottery. I attend parent council and church meetings, watching from the sidelines, reluctant to volunteer.

One of my husband's co-workers gave him the name of a prominent psychiatrist. He had nothing but praise for this young man who had helped his wife with her depression. I told my husband that I wasn't depressed, but I did write down the doctor's name. That was three years ago.

I did some research on the internet about depression. Modern treatments seem to be very beneficial to many, without any catastrophic side effects. Sometimes just talking to someone can help. I wish that someone could reassure me that this could happen with me. I dread the thought of taking pills. I won't even take an aspirin if I have a headache. So as tempted as I am to make an appointment with this psychiatrist, there is always something that holds me back.

The girls are too preoccupied with their own lives to notice that I am becoming more and more quiet and that I have perfected the art of maintaining a plastic smile. My husband appears married to his business, and feels that extravagant gifts and luxury cruises compensate for his lack of attentiveness towards me.

I decided to submit this and I hope that I may find a solution to this sadness by reading the stories written by others. Maybe there are other women out there who feel sad and don't know why either. Maybe some of them have taken that big step and had the courage to ask for help. Right now, I'm still,

Sad in the Suberbs

*****

I have cancer. The doctor wants to remove a breast. Nobody else in my family ever had cancer. They all tiptoe around me like I might be contagious. They don't want to talk about it.

I look at myself in the mirror. I remember being a child and wishing I had breasts. When they started to develop I was so excited. Now maybe boys would be interested in me.

But then I got tired of wearing a bra all the time. I longed to throw them all away and have my childhood body back again.

But instead I married a wonderful man who admired my breasts, but really was more in love with what was inside, in my heart. He loves to tease my nipples with his fingers or his tongue. He loves to suck on them just as my babies had done.

But now there is going to be one less to suck on. Oh, I know all about that surgery where they rebuild a breast and nipple. But we aren't millionaires and our health insurance won't cover it.

The doctor told me I'd have to come to the hospital for treatments after the surgery. He warned me about the nasty side effects. I don't want to be nauseous and lose my hair. Isn't it bad enough that I will only have one breast instead of two?

And then there's the part about the low energy level. Who will chase after my three young sons? The twins just turned two, and their big brother is only three.

I used to take so many things for granted. I should have enjoyed that freedom more when I still had it. Now I have to learn to be dependent on others, and even then I may still die.

Things will never be the same again. I have cancer.

*****

I once was happy,
I once was free,
But now I'm not
Who I used to be.

18

So many changes
Are happening in my life
Times are so confusing
I don't want to be a wife.

I hate to cook
I hate to clean
I hate to dust
And I can always tell where he's been
.

He leaves a trail
And I can always tell
What he's worn, what he eats
God, my life is hell.

I finally sit down
I try to relax
When I suddenly remember
About his slacks.

I race to the dryer
Open the door and frown
His slacks are full of wrinkles
And so is my nightgown.

He always complains
That I never do anything right
It seems like since we got married
All we do is fight.

We never go out
We never have fun
Dating was sure different
I want to just run.

*****

Contributors' Stories Part 2: Anxiety

My husband, sons and I moved to Winnipeg from Montreal two years ago. I started having panic attacks three years ago when our daughter was killed in a car accident. It was a terrible shock to all of us. She was only eight and had gone out to a friend's summer house for the weekend. On the way home, a drunk driver crossed the centre line and hit the car she was traveling in. Everyone in the car was killed. Only the drunk driver survived.

Before her death, I drove my three kids everywhere. I drove to shopping malls, the spa, the hairdresser, medical appointments and countless other destinations. I was never afraid to drive. And now, whenever I get behind the wheel, and sometimes when I'm just a passenger, I have these attacks. Whenever I hear about drunk drivers I have attacks.

My heart starts to race, I have trouble breathing and I feel nauseous. I hate when this happens. My doctor in Montreal gave me valium. I soon became addicted to this drug.

My husband was offered a promotion if we moved to Winnipeg. I had hoped that once we moved, the attacks would go away. I also wanted to get off the Valium.

I couldn't believe it when I was told that there were no family practitioners in our area who were taking new patients at the time we arrived in Winnipeg. I used to think Montreal healthcare was inferior to other provinces but this situation was quite upsetting. One of the men my husband works with pulled some strings and was able to get us in to see his cousin's neighbor. I was then told that the wait for a psychiatrist was several months. I was ready to go back to Montreal at this point.

We have lived in Vancouver, Calgary, Regina and Montreal. I have never before had such a terrible experience in obtaining healthcare.

I finally did get in to see a psychiatrist. I was weaned off the valium and was given medication for anxiety. Clonazepam is a pill that has helped to calm me down considerably. I take my pills and see my therapist regularly. The attacks are not as frequent or as intense now.

I miss my little girl and think of her everyday. I wonder what she would be doing now if she were still alive. She'd be eleven now. She had the cutest smile and beautiful blue eyes. These memories are actually comforting now. Grieving takes time.

*****

I was standing in line at Sobey's with my groceries when I had my first panic attack. I remember abandoning my shopping cart and racing outside. I couldn't breathe. I needed fresh air. I collapsed on the sidewalk, doubling over in pain. I was sure I was having a heart attack. Meanwhile, one of the staff at Sobey's had called 911 and another one sat with me until the ambulance arrived.

I felt like a complete idiot when the paramedics arrived. By that time the attack had passed and I felt perfectly normal. They insisted on checking me over anyways. Everyone around me had been convinced that I was having a heart attack.

That was four years ago. I still have the odd attack, but not very often. I now have medication. I know that certain things can trigger these attacks. I try to avoid these situations. Psychotherapy has really helped me too.

*****

I used to shake constantly. I didn't trust myself to carry a cup of coffee from the kitchen to the living room. I dropped books and pens and

22

other things I tried to carry. I noticed that people were staring at me but were too polite to say anything.

I became so uncomfortable that I avoided going out unless I had to. If I had to go grocery shopping it became a major production. I missed parties and concerts and became somewhat of a recluse.

I was so miserable and unhappy all the time. I finally got up the nerve to go and see my doctor.

That was almost a year ago. At first I tried Wellbutrin, but I gained weight. Then I tried Celexa and my sex drive disappeared along with the shakes. I'm now on Paxil and have been on the same dosage for quite a while.

I have also been on a tranquilizer called Clonazepam that calms me down and helps me sleep.

I'm not afraid to go out anymore. And the shakes have all but disappeared. I feel like *ME* again.

*****

I'm a chemist conducting research for a private company. This type of work demands a steady and calm hand as I handle various chemicals and glass apparatus. I enjoy this job as I have free reign and I'm on my own schedule most of the time.

I returned from holidays to find that an assistant had been hired to help me with my research. At first I thought this was a good idea, as she could do more of the tedious work involved. This would free me up to experiment more on my own. And I must admit I looked forward to having someone to clean up after me.

It turns out that this assistant was the CEO's ex-wife. Apparently one of the divorce clauses guaranteed her a position with the company indefinitely and it also promised a promotion after one year.

I had taken for granted my job stability. The only promotion this woman could have was to assume my position. Where would that leave me?

The shaking began about that time. I trembled on the job, often spilling powders and dropping test-tubes. I'd accidentally hit the wrong button on the computer and would have to repeat tests over and over again. The shaking got worse and affected me at home. I began to dread going to work. I wanted to just stay in bed all day and sleep. But I was too jittery to sleep.

I used to enjoy my job. I now hated it. I used to be very outgoing and sociable. I was now quiet and morose. I knew that I had to do something. But making a decision was just too overwhelming for me to even consider.

One Monday, I dragged myself out of bed and headed to work. To my surprise, the lab was still locked and my assistant was nowhere to be found. Now I really started to worry. What if she had decided to complain about the problems I was having in the lab? After all, time and supplies were being wasted.

Lost in my thoughts, I didn't even hear the head of human resources enter the room. He cleared his throat rather noisily and that got my attention. I was shocked at what he had to say. Apparently my assistant had eloped with her lawyer over the weekend and was not the least bit interested in working anymore.

The lab was mine again! The shaking and trembling stopped almost immediately. A feeling of relief came over me. My job was secure. My assistant was merely a bad dream. I was awake now and had only good things to look forward to.

I was lucky. My anxiety went away without any therapy or drugs. It was an eye-opener to see how circumstances could affect my body and my performance at work. I then thought about how many people are forced to work at jobs they hate because they need the money. I wonder how many of them are receiving treatment for anxiety.

*****

Contributors' Stories Part 3: Post Traumatic Stress Disorder

My dad was killed in New York in 9-11. The company he worked for had its corporate headquarters there. I stayed glued to the TV, hoping that I'd recognize my dad as one of the survivors. My mom kept checking the hospitals. And the company here in Toronto was doing all they could.

It just seemed too surreal. This couldn't be happening. It was a horrible disaster for the Americans, but people didn't realize how terrible it was for Canadians as well. My mom was devastated. As an only child, she became very overprotective of me.

The years have passed and we have both gone for therapy to help us cope. My mom seems to be doing ok. She went back to teaching and it keeps her busy. At first the kids asked her all kinds of questions. She found that talking about my dad to them has helped her to heal.

I'm still a mess. I cringe when the annual Father And Son Dinner is held at my school, even though my uncles are all eager to fill in. Father's Day gatherings are the toughest. All my cousins and friends have their dads with them, but I don't.

I miss him so much. We used to toss around a football or a baseball. He was going to put up a basketball hoop in our driveway. I remember how we used to tent out in our backyard in the summer. All these memories make me cry.

One day I saw a quote in a magazine I was reading. It said: Don't cry because it's over. Smile because it happened. That has now become my motto. Instead of crying over the memories, I try to smile at the memories.

I still feel sad because my dad died when I was only nine, but I sure was lucky to have him all those years.

My psychologist and I talk a lot about that. He says I've come a long way. Maybe I have. But I still feel down, and cheated out of a great person who should still be around.

*****

I am a survivor of the Holocaust. The number tattooed on my arm will be there until I die. The atrocities committed by the Nazis are too heinous to print. They roll through my mind in the form of nightmares. I wake up and my heart is racing and I check to see that I really am in my own bed in my own apartment. I always sleep with a light on.

There have been articles in the newspaper and on the internet about people who do not believe that a Holocaust actually occurred. My doctor tells me that denial is a common defense mechanism. I shake my head and wonder about these people.

I lost my entire family during the war. My parents and my brothers were herded onto a cattle car in the railroad station. I came home from a friend's to find our house empty and furniture and other items broken and thrown around.

I wanted to go back to my friend's house, but I had just made it home before curfew. I didn't dare go out and I was terrified at staying alone all night by myself.

The next morning I tried to make my way to my friend's house. The Germans had continued their raids in other neighborhoods, and somehow I knew that I would never again see my family or my friend again.

It was almost a relief when the Germans found me and took me away in a truck. From there I was transferred to a train and my final destination was a concentration camp.

When I was liberated from this camp at the end of the war, physically I was a mere skeleton of my former self. My mind has never been the same since.

I survived, supposedly one of the lucky ones. My life has been a struggle. I have never married and I keep to myself a lot. But when I read about these people who believe that there never was a Holocaust, I feel angry.

I am a human being, but never was given the opportunity to do anything with my life until I was much older. By then I didn't want an education. I have been blind in one eye and had all my fingernails pulled out. I had toes cut off, and damage was done to my kidneys and bladder. And those are just the signs of some of the abuse I endured in the hands of the Nazis. There was more, much more.

I feel the tears coming. Please print this in your book. The message must get out to everyone that the Holocaust was very real and that it did happen.

*****

I just got back from an extended tour of duty in Afghanistan. I knew that when I signed up for the army I'd be training and working away from home. I didn't realize just how hard it was going to be on my wife and kids. We all missed each other but then we all just took for granted that I'd be home after about 6 months and would hopefully remain there for quite a while before being sent out on another tour.

I had only been home for a few days when I got the call that I was to be ready to fly overseas in two days. I was not told how long I would be gone for nor where I was going. This meant only one thing....... that I was headed somewhere in Afghanistan. This mission could mean life or death. Neither my wife nor I had any family in Winnipeg. Our families were all back home in the Maritimes.

We were all crying when it was time for me to leave. I took one last look at my daughters, ages five and six. I'd be missing some real important times with them growing up. As for my wife, we were high school sweethearts and had only been married for a little over seven years.

When I finally did come home several months later, I just couldn't believe how everything had changed so much. My family seemed like strangers to me. The girls had grown taller and were lots mouthier. My wife introduced me to my son who had been conceived on my last visit home. He clung to his mom and screamed every time I tried to go near him.

The kids were all in bed when my wife and I finally had some time together. I suggested we go to bed early. I longed to hold her in my arms again and show her how much I had missed her and how much I loved her. Instead she just wanted to talk.

She told me how lonely and scared she was after I left. She told me how the girls cried and fought all the time. She felt so tired all the time and finally went to the doctor so that he could confirm what she already knew. She was pregnant. She toyed with the idea of going back to the Maritimes to be with her family. But she didn't have the money. She cried a lot, yelled at the girls, and couldn't have cared less when they began using bad language they picked up from the kids at school. After a horrible pregnancy, labor and delivery, her reward was a colicky baby. The girls came down with chicken pox shortly after the baby was born. The baby didn't develop the same way the girls had. He didn't respond the same way. He fussed and screamed a lot. Her pediatrician sent her to a specialist, where it was discovered that the baby was deaf and blind in one eye.

At first I didn't know how to respond. This wasn't the welcome home I'd expected to receive. I had expected being up all night making love to my wife. I thought the girls would be so excited that their dad was home. I knew that a son had been born while I was away. I just couldn't handle all this now.

For months I had lived in the streets or the shelter of trees or a rock crevice. The first time I had a proper shower and shave and haircut was the day before I came home. I had to borrow a toothbrush as I had lost mine long ago. I slept always on the alert. And I don't think that I always counted on that being sleep. My body was swollen from bug bites and there were poisonous snakes to watch out for. I watched my buddies die in action. I was wounded myself, followed by infection and high fever. I saw guys go home, missing an arm or a leg or paralyzed. I can still smell the smoke from the bombs and the guns. I can still hear the gunfire and the approaching bombers. I narrowly missed being taken a prisoner on several occasions. I killed men I didn't even know. The only reason was that if I didn't kill them first, they would surely kill me. I had been living in hell defending my country.

Things were feeling very strange those next few days. I got real compulsive that the house had to be clean all the time. The girls were annoyed because they had gotten used to living in a messy home. And watching my son sit in a playpen and hardly move all day was too overwhelming. My wife found every excuse not to be around me. She had to go shopping, she had to do something with the girls, she had to get her hair cut, and then I found out about the biggest excuse of all.

She was seeing another man. It had started a couple of months after I left. He was there for her through the pregnancy. He was her labor coach. He tracked down the specialist for my son. Hell, maybe he was even the boy's father, though she denies this.

We went for counseling, but we both knew in our hearts that our marriage was over. I still wake up shaking in the middle of the night. Loud noises still bother me. I'm taking all kinds of pills now. I haven't seen the girls in months. My wife called the other day and said she wanted to marry this man so we'd have to get our divorce done faster. She was pregnant again.

Yep, I got a real hero's welcome allright. I had no idea that my life was going to change so much over a period of three years. I take my pills, I cry a lot, I go out the odd time, usually to the grocery store and medical appointments only. My doctor says that it will become easier over time. I guess I just have to believe him. I had to take a leave of absence from work. I wish the nightmares would stop and that I'd feel safe again. Right now I just want to be by myself. My family offered to come from the Maritimes. I said no. They offered to fly me home. I said no. After all the noise and all the fighting in the war, I just want peace and quiet.

*****

We lived out on a farm in Saskatchewan. There was my Mom, Dad and my three younger brothers and me. We were a happy and close family until the summer I turned fifteen.

That summer it rained way too much and the fields got flooded. I remember going out to the tractor with my Mom and brothers and trying to get it unstuck in all that mud. The water was over our rubber boots and we got all soaked and muddy. The whole time we were struggling, my Dad sat in his rocking chair in the house, puffing on his

29

pipe. We all pleaded with him to help us, but he just ignored us. After what seemed like hours, we gave up on the tractor and came back into the house.

My Mom told us four kids to go on upstairs and clean ourselves up. I think she just wanted to be alone with my Dad. Even with the water running, we could all hear her harsh voice screaming at my Dad. Once we were all cleaned up we were all scared to go downstairs. All of a sudden it got real quiet down there.

We waited some and then quietly came down the staircase. My Dad was still puffing away on his pipe and rocking in his chair. My Mom was sitting at the kitchen table, shaking and trying to drink a cup of tea. She looked real angry. Her face was all red and it looked like she'd been crying.

Mom looked up at us and yelled for us to go upstairs and get ready for bed. We were surprised. It was only three in the afternoon. We hadn't eaten since breakfast that day and our tummies were growling. But when Mom was in one of her moods, we didn't dare disobey. So up we went.

The four of us ransacked our bedrooms to find some leftover snacks. All we found were some peanuts and bubble gum. To pass the time and try to forget how hungry we were, we played checkers.

From time to time we heard Mom and Dad yelling at each other. Actually, it sounded like Mom was doing most of the yelling. We covered our ears with our pillows to drown out the noise and finally went to bed crying.

The more it rained that summer the worse it got. Dad never moved out of his chair. He wouldn't talk to any of us. He just smoked, rocked and slept in his chair. He smelled awful because he wouldn't take a bath and never changed his clothes. He looked awful and didn't comb his hair or shave.

The only time Mom talked to us was to call us to the table for meals or to tell us to do our laundry. And she would scream at us if we forgot to do our chores around the house. But at least she had stopped yelling at Dad.

Just before school started, my Mom told us that our grandparents were coming to visit from Ontario, and that they were taking us four boys back home with them. She told us to pack up our clothes and any books or games we wanted to take with us.

I'm almost thirty now, and with the help of a loving wife I am trying to heal. You see, after us kids went to live with our grandparents, my Mom burned the house down with my Dad still sleeping in his rocking chair. She's still in jail, and none of us kids have heard from her or seen her since.

My wife and I go to weekly sessions with a therapist. He tells us that depression is a silent killer. He says that my brothers and I were not in any way to blame for what happened at home. He said we need to move on, and although I will never forget the past, I sure don't want things to turn out that way when my wife and I have a family of our own.

My youngest brother committed suicide a few years ago after several attempts. My other two brothers became alcoholics and died in a car accident last year. And yes, they were to blame for the accident. They wrapped their car around a tree in their drunken state. The only other victim was the tree.

I cry a lot. There was no reason for my brothers to die.

Thank God I have the support of my wife and her family, my therapist, and a few close friends. My grandparents were wonderful to us kids, and they are now living in a nursing home close by, so we do see them quite often.

That's my story.

*****

I live just southwest of Winnipeg. I have been here since Hurricane Katrina destroyed my home and killed many of my relatives and friends. One minute my life was so normal. I'd wait for my children to board the school bus and then I'd drive to work. But when Katrina came along the nightmare began for me and my family.

My mother and father were killed when the roof of a shopping centre collapsed. They had sought shelter from the storm in there, along with hundreds of others. My husband was a school teacher. He saved many children from dying as the school had a shelter that by some miracle did not flood. My husband died when a large piece of glass flew through the air and literally sliced his body into two pieces.

The building where I worked was very new. There was a storm shelter that had minimal flooding. My colleagues and I all survived thanks to that shelter. The telephone lines were down and there was no electricity. When we were finally allowed to exit the building I was shocked by all the destruction and debris. I found my car upside-down several blocks from where I had parked it. I saw dogs and cats high up in trees. Blood was everywhere. People were screaming for help. Children were crying. I still have nightmares and see all this.

I would walk down a street where one or two houses were left standing while the rest had been destroyed. There was water everywhere, deeper and muddier in some areas than in others. I vomited when I reached what should have been my house. There was no sign of my babysitter or my two year old son. I sat down on the ground and cried and cried.

The next thing I remember is waking up in a hospital where I was reunited with my son. By some miracle God had spared his life. The babysitter was not as fortunate. I looked at myself in the mirror and saw a very disheveled woman with a bandage on her face. I had aged twenty years. The doctor told me that the cut on my face had required twenty stitches. My son had a few bruises, but other than that he was ok. In the aftermath and chaos that followed I learned of my husband's death. It took several days before I found my two daughters who had remained in their school.

The stories everyone told were gruesome and frightening. I feared that my children would never be happy and carefree again. And I prayed that my baby son would not remember any of this when he was older.

Despite the looting that went on, many people were kind and generous. We were never thirsty or hungry, but I knew that we had to get away from here. There was nothing left for us. We were fortunate to be alive and to have the clothes on our backs. I remembered that my cousin had married a Canadian a few years back. The Red Cross helped me to locate her. She insisted that we all come to live with her. I thought she was living in Minnesota, but it turns out that they moved to Manitoba when her husband finished school.

The years have passed but we all still have trouble sleeping and have nightmares. I consider us the lucky ones. We survived a horrible natural disaster and were able to go somewhere to heal. Our Canadian relatives helped us settle in and adjust to rural live in Manitoba. My son doesn't remember much. My girls and I have been going for therapy. The doctor at first gave us pills to calm us down. We still see a psychologist regularly and I encourage my daughters to talk. When the skies cloud over and it rains, we still feel tense.

Last summer there was a big tornado in Elie. I really feel badly for the people from that town. I could really relate to their fears and troubles. And I was very surprised that many chose to stay in Elie and rebuild their lives.

For the time being we will remain here and heal. My faith in God has grown stronger. My children never complain about attending church every Sunday. All I dream about for us is to have a safe and secure home and that we are all together. Material things are not what matters in life. We need to appreciate every single day because we never know if this day will be the last one.

*****

I work as interpreter in hospital. I myself have been in Canada 3 years so my English not so good. The other day patient comes to hospital and she talks Farsi. One of the languages I know is Farsi. I stayed with lady while she was admitted and left when lots of family came.

The next day I come to visit. Lady looked so sad and not happy. But in her eyes was anger. We started to talk together. She complained about hospital. She not like food. She not like room. Too small and three others in it. Family can come only at certain times. She cries and says if she were back home in Iran family would take care and not need hospital. She is very mad at Canadian soldiers. She loves her country, but the soldiers make it dangerous. She would like to die and not stay in Canada. Her husband is back home. She worries she will not see him anymore. Children came to Canada with her. Have no father to keep them obedient and they are wild like Canadian children. Schools here are bad. Girls must stay home and clean and cook. Girls need to go and shop but should not be alone. Bad things will happen.

She blames wars in Iran, Iraq, Afghanistan......everywhere Canadian soldiers to blame. She mad that yellow ribbons honor soldiers here and newspapers honor soldiers like heroes.

Lady speaks no English and tells children to speak Farsi at home. Children not to forget their language and homeland. Children like this city. They want to stay. Lady not understand why children shoot guns at school or have knives. No war here like at home. She say boys and girls need to learn like army. This real life. Don't teach this at Canada schools.

Lady say a story two sides. She say it important people hear her side.

*****

I grew up in Thompson, Manitoba. I was the only girl in the family and had two younger brothers. My parents were both social workers. Oh, did I mention that we were white and not aboriginal like most of the people who live up there? My parents thought it would be a great experience for them to work up north for a few years. The problem is that when I was born, they never moved back to Winnipeg like they were supposed to.

Those native girls were a bunch of whores. They smoked, drank, sniffed, screwed anything in sight, got pregnant, had abortions, or tried to pass the baby off to their families to raise. Like that would do any good! Most of them had only one parent, who was usually as messed up as they were.

The native boys were obnoxious too. They reeked of booze and solvent and all they ever thought about was getting laid. They used to taunt and tease the girls, especially me because I was white. Funny that two social workers were too blind to see what was going on in their own family.

I was fourteen when all hell broke loose. Some older boys followed me home one day after school. I told them to get lost and fled to the safety of my house. My parents were at work and my brothers were out. I smiled at the thought of having the entire place to myself. I grabbed a bag of chips and planted myself down in front of the tv. I was just dozing off when I heard a loud crash and the sound of glass breaking. The next thing I knew, those guys who had followed me home were all over me. I screamed, I kicked and I fought as hard as I could. But there were six of them and only one of me. I was only fourteen and still a virgin. They all laughed and said it was time for my initiation. A couple of them held me down and they all took turns raping me. It hurt so much and I was crying my heart out. After what seemed like hours to me, my brothers came home.

The older guys grabbed them and made them watch what was going on. I was so humiliated I just wanted to die right then and there. And if that wasn't bad enough, they forced my brothers to touch me all over. Then they started fooling around with my brothers too. They even tried to make one of them put his penis in my mouth. I think that was when I passed out.

When I came to, my brothers were crying. They thought I was dead! The older guys had all left by then. One of my brothers had covered me with a blanket and the other one had phoned my parents at work.

The best is yet to come. Instead of sympathizing with me over the violent attack, my parents concluded that I must have been flirting with these guys. I couldn't believe my ears! Not to mention that my brothers were very upset by what they had seen and what they had been forced to do.

I'm twenty-two now and I'm living with a cousin in an apartment in Winnipeg. I've never gotten over what happened that day. My parents wanted to hush it all up and wouldn't take me to the doctor or for counseling. They told me and my brothers that we should forget about what happened and never talk about it with anyone. So that was what we did. My cousin and I have shared this apartment for a couple of years now, and she doesn't even know about this.

I hope that one day I'll have the courage to talk to somebody about this. I hope my story gets into your book. I bet I'm not the only one out there that has been gang-banged. And I like the idea that I didn't have to tell you my name or anything.

One good thing I can say about my social worker parents is that we did leave Thompson at the end of that school year. As soon as I could afford to move out, I moved in with my cousin. I have cut off all ties with my parents.

I work in an office as a receptionist. I still freak whenever I see an aboriginal guy. I just shake and want to cry. I've never had a boyfriend. I'm scared to go out on a date, even.

I may be twenty-two now, but in my heart I often wonder what happened to that innocent little fourteen-year-old girl. Life has just never been the same since I was raped.

*****

When I was growing up I was an only child. My parents were overprotective, especially my mother. The other kids used to tease me because I wasn't allowed to walk to school, play on sports teams, or even use some of the playground equipment. It eased off a little in high school, but I was the last one of all my friends to get a driver's license.

I got a scholarship to a university in another province. I really wanted to get away where nobody knew me and I could make a fresh start. My parents weren't happy, but they gave in and let me go. Thankfully no-one that I had grown up with was at this university.

I had to room with 2 other boys in the dorm. I thought they were really cool, and the kind of guys I had always wanted to be. They drank beer, smoked pot, and always had girls coming around. Interestingly enough, they never teased me when I told them why I wanted to get away from home. I thought these guys were real pals. That first year was a great one and we all decided to room together in the fall.

Somehow things seemed a little different when we got back to classes in the fall. They still included me in a lot of things like usual, but they were often whispering and I couldn't hear what they were saying. One day they asked me if I had ever used a gun. I was totally shocked. Of course I had never used a gun! Why would I?

They then told me that they had gotten together over the summer and had participated in a little robbery spree when they had found a gun in a garbage can. They said they had never actually fired the gun. All they ever stole was cigarettes and some small electronic stuff. I was horrified!

They then told me they were planning to rob an arcade and wanted to know if I was interested. When I hesitated to answer, they taunted me and told me I was just a chicken and that they'd make my life really miserable if I didn't agree to help them. I knew they meant it. They were really the only close friends I'd ever had, and I didn't want that to change. And I knew that they were capable of harassing me all the time, so I agreed to go with them.

What a mistake that was! A silent alarm was tripped at the arcade when we broke in. The cops were there in minutes. Here I was, holding a gun, while the other two got away. The cops slapped some handcuffs on me after they got the gun, and then they shoved me into a squad car and took me to the station for questioning.

I told them about the other two. The cops found them back in our dorm room, studying. That really made me suspicious. Those two never studied. Somehow they always managed to get tests ahead of time and they always bullied some smart kid into writing their term papers.

The problems started when the cops chose not to believe me. They said my friends claimed that I had threatened them with a gun and that's why they had broken in. They ran off when the cops came because they were scared I might shoot them. They must have put on quite a performance.

The cops charged me and kept me in jail, and my two so-called friends walked. The charges stuck, but fortunately I was given a suspended sentence and probation. There had been no bullets in the gun. The university expelled me and I returned home.

I wish I could get even with those two lowlifes. My parents are worse than ever. The neighbors are gossiping about me. I can't go back to school for a while. I wish I still had that gun. I'd get some bullets and I swear I'd learn how to use that gun.

$$*****$$

I am forty-two years old now and my life is a mess. It just gradually got worse and worse. Finally I broke down and went to talk to a counselor at work. I am so glad that I did. She has been a tremendous help to me. Maybe now things will be better.

I was the only boy in my family and had two older sisters. Not only were they blonde and beautiful, but they were also identical twins. What an attraction that was! I'm two years younger, but all anyone ever talked about was the twins. We'd get together on the holidays with the rest of the family and I'd be totally ignored. When I started kindergarten they were in grade two. That meant that we rode the same bus to school everyday. They would immediately race to the back of the bus and I always felt like I was invisible. If I came anywhere near them they told me to get lost. Of course this made all the other kids laugh at me and tease me. It didn't matter how hard I tried, I just couldn't make any friends.

All through elementary school, I was always the last one to be picked for a sports team, or to work with on a project. I felt like a square peg that was trying to fit into a round hole. I was very lonely and spent a lot of time at home by myself.

Things weren't much better in middle school or in high school. The other kids just seemed to get meaner and meaner. They'd grab my baseball cap off my head and toss it around until they found some mud or water for it to land in. They'd throw my books out the open windows of the bus. They even locked me in the janitor's closet at school for a whole afternoon.

My sisters treated me like I was some contagious disease. They were so popular and had so many friends. They were invited to lots of parties and guys were always asking them out on dates. They told me I was weird and that I should never talk to them in public. Of course, in front of my parents it was a whole different story. They always fussed over me.

The counselor explained to me that I had been bullied for many years. Today there are programs in schools so that staff and students alike are aware of the behaviors and the consequences. Back then there was nothing. I didn't dare report anyone because then they'd just make my life even more miserable. I'd often tell the teachers that I had lost or forgotten a book at home.

Because I had been bullied so much it affected my career plans. After I graduated high school, I worked for a small construction company. After a year, I left as the company was placed in receivership and my job was eliminated.

I took a course at a technical school and became a car mechanic. I worked on my own and nobody bothered me. I never went to any of the social functions and wasn't the friendliest person in the world.

I was very shy around women and people often thought I was gay. I was just socially totally backwards. I never dated much, but by some miracle I actually got married when I was in my thirties. We hadn't been married long when my wife confided in me that the only reason she married me was that she knew I could support her and she wouldn't have to work. She then went on to tell me that there would always be other men in her life as I wasn't enough of a man for her.

I lived with this for almost five years. One day I came home from work and found a note on the table. She had run off with another guy and was filing for a divorce. She just wanted to get rid of me so that she could finally live a better life.

The counselor has worked with me in improving my social skills and in asserting myself. She explained how my sisters were spoiled and selfish. It wasn't my fault that they and the rest of the kids at school didn't want to be around me. She also remarked that my parents and teachers never noticed how unhappy I was. She kept impressing upon me that I had done nothing wrong. I was just a really sensitive guy. Someday I might find a woman who would appreciate that quality.

Bullying. It's a very common issue that people talk about today. There are even tv commercials and newspaper ads. The schools and community clubs often have speakers come out to talk to parents. The kids talk about it at school.

I only wish some of these resources had been around when I was growing up.

*****

Contributors' Stories Part 4: Seasonal Affective Disorder

I suffer from Seasonal Affective Disorder. Much as I detest labels, I am glad that my condition finally has a name. And I know now that there are things I can do so that my life isn't always so dreary.

I was sitting at home feeling sorry for myself when one of those boring talk shows came on. They were all usually about dieting, hairstyles, fashion, pets, relationships, and were always so predictable. The guest on this show was a young man in his mid-thirties. I really found myself listening to what he was saying. And suddenly everything made sense.

He said he felt like a mole in the winter. He'd get up in the morning and it was still dark outside when he went to work. He did something with computers and was cooped up in an office building all day. When it was time to drive home, it was dark outside again. Boy, could I ever associate with that!

He didn't have any energy left by the time he got home and he never felt like eating a proper dinner. Instead he'd snack on chips and other junk foods while watching TV. I looked down at my jelly beans and jujubes.

So I wasn't the only one out there with these symptoms. That was a little reassuring.

He then went on to say that he made an appointment with his doctor. He was told to go for short brisk walks twice a day. To get his diet back on track to healthier foods, he was told to purchase cut up vegetables and fruits at the grocery store for snacks. He was told all about healthy prepared foods that were available for meals and required little effort. This was really starting to sound good.

He then was advised to buy special fluorescent light bulbs to install in his office. These had the effect of a more natural daylight rather than a harsh indoor light. Wouldn't you know it? I work in a cubicle with a desk lamp. But, wait! He said that these same lights were available as a desk lamp. This would work in my office. Because it was portable, I could get one for home and take it from room to room.

I was so excited that I couldn't wait for the program to end. Here it was, 8:30 at night, and I was determined to start my search for these special lights. I grabbed my keys and raced to my car. I forgot all about how dark it was outside as I went from store to store to find the perfect lamp. With that out of the way I then went grocery shopping. I picked up vegetable and fruit trays. I picked up cooked chicken and roasts that just had to be reheated. I picked up frozen veggies that take only minutes to micro.

By the time I got home it was way later than I usually stay up, and I was exhausted. I hurriedly stored the food away. I set up one of the lamps on my nightstand, turned it on and settled into bed with a book. I then set my alarm clock for a half hour earlier so that I could sit by the lamp and have a leisurely breakfast the next day.

The next morning I actually packed a lunch and made a point of leaving the office and going for a walk.

Life isn't so SAD anymore.

*****

In the fall the trees shed their leaves and the flowers die. Then the winter comes and brings more doom and gloom. I feel like I'm living underground. I take a bus to work in the dark. I have a small cubicle at work. I eat my lunch at my desk usually. I go home in the dark. It's like I never see the sun. And I think maybe I'll never see the sun again ever.

I don't want to go out anywhere. Heavy boots and coats weigh me down even more. Some days it's so cold out it's hard to breathe. It's just too much effort to go out to the bar or to a gym. And of course the days when I don't work it's usually stormy so there's no sun then either. Maybe I'll win a lottery and I'll move to somewhere that's warm and sunny the whole year round. Then I won't waste half the year with no energy and feeling listless all the time.

*****

I think I need to move to California. Whenever I visit my friends down there I feel so much better. It's warm, the sun shines a lot, flowers grow year round, and there is no snow or freezing rain. I wouldn't have to bus it to work in the dark and then bus it home in the dark.

I have so much more energy when I'm down there. It's no big deal to come home from work and then go out again and meet someone for coffee. And it doesn't matter what time I come and go. I can still smell the fragrance of the flowers and wear a light jacket and sandals instead of a parka and boots.

I spent five months down south doing some research for a Canadian company. That's how I know how much better I feel in that climate. I have been going back to visit friends for a month every winter since then. And it's so horrible when it's time to come back to the snow and bitter cold when my holiday is over.

I usually put on weight over the winter. I prefer to sit at home and watch movies rather than jog or walk outside. I did try joining a fitness centre, but I didn't have the energy to go there very often. Somehow it's a lot more cozy to put on a pair of flannel pj's and wrap up in a cuddly afghan and stay in on weeknights.

I really think I need to move to California. Then I could throw away my heavy coats and jackets, my boots, gloves, hats and scarves. I wouldn't need a snow shovel and I could walk out onto a patio all winter long without wrapping up in a blanket.

I really think I need to move to California sooner than later.

*****

Winnipeg is the most awful city to live in. When it's summer the mosquitoes and the wasps get you. Fall is depressing. The flowers die. The trees lose their leaves. And it always snows before Halloween. And

43

then the streets are so slippery and full of snow. I hate driving in the winter. It's dark when you get up in the morning and it's dark when I get home from school. And it's always freezing outside. We get freezing rain in the spring. That's even more of a nuisance than the hail we get in the summer. And now there's all these tornadoes happening too.

Some days I like to just stay in bed and sleep. It's too hard to go outside. The school can get a substitute for me. Everyone likes first-graders. They're cute and they think teachers are gods. Wait until they get a little older!

I like painting and I go to art classes. But not in the winter. It takes too much of an effort to drive to the church. It's only two blocks from my house, but I won't walk outside in the winter.

I absolutely hate going shopping in the winter. The shopping carts get stuck in the ruts in parking lots. The winds are bitter. I don't have a garage so it means cleaning my car off for a change. I don't like scraping ice and clearing off snow. And the car is so cold inside until it warms up. And then I have to carry in all the groceries and put them away. I'm too exhausted from being outside.

I like Christmas. But I don't go to many parties or dinners. It's too cold outside to dress up in holiday clothes. It's much cozier to snuggle in bed at home.

I sometimes wonder why I stay here. I have no family here. They're all dead. I have friends, but I can make friends anywhere. I don't think I'd be better off anywhere else in Canada. The provinces on the coasts get way too much rain. I actually heard that Winnipeg has the greatest number of hours of sunshine. So there's no point moving.

Every fall I feel worse and worse. Every winter gets worse and worse. I'm having a checkup later this month. Maybe my doctor will have a solution.

*****

Contributors' Stories Part 5: Post Partum Depression

I was so excited when I found out I was pregnant! My husband and I were like two little kids in a candy store. Did we ever shop in anticipation of our first little one to arrive!

We put in new carpeting and new wallpaper and new curtains in the spare room that was now to be the nursery. Everything coordinated from the light switch on the wall (it had a dimmer too) down to the comforter and bumper pads. The sheet sets were muted shades of purple, green, and orange to accent the color scheme we had chosen for the room. We painted stars on the ceiling and the light fixture looked like the moon with a big smiley face on it. We found a beautiful rocking chair to match the crib, change table, and dressers. We bought these cute little hangers with animals on them to hang in the closet. We bought a vaporizer and tucked it away in a closet should we ever need it.

I went shopping with my Mom and we bought lotions, powders, shampoos, soaps, and of course Vaseline. We bought boxes full of colorful disposable diapers, teeny tiny facecloths, and darling hooded bath towels. We bought a baby bathtub with a lounger in it.

Meanwhile my husband installed an infant seat in my car. He also bought some children's music on a cd to play while we were on the road. He bought a lightweight folding stroller for traveling and an English pram to use while at home.

My sisters and I went shopping for little t-shirts and sleepers. And of course a monstrous diaper bag to carry all the supplies that would be needed.

My co-workers threw a baby shower for me and I have never seen so many Fisher Price toys and stuffed animals in one room in my life!

I went to all my scheduled doctor appointments, treasured the little sonogram pictures, ate a healthy diet, and made sure to exercise. We attended pre-natal classes and my loving husband was such a wonderful coach.

As my pregnancy progressed, I lost my figure and turned into a big blob. But it just felt so great when the baby kicked or moved. I sat in the rocker and read stories to my little one and sang songs. I had my bag for the hospital packed well ahead of time. Once, I glanced out the window and saw two of my girlfriends wheeling their babies to the park. Soon that would be me!

My in-laws owned a restaurant and they stocked my freezer so that I wouldn't have to cook for a year! Our baby was to be the first grandchild on both sides of the family, and would this one ever be spoiled by everyone!

The big day finally arrived. My waters broke and the labor pains began in the middle of the night. I timed the contractions and knew that I had a long way to go yet. I was deliriously happy! I watched my husband sleep and felt like I was the luckiest woman in the whole wide world.

It was almost noon and the contractions were becoming more intense and more often. Time to wake up sleepyhead. He went from a state of grogginess to panic in a matter of seconds. He dressed quickly, grabbed my bag, and with the other hand he guided me so gently towards the car. I called my doctor on my cell and told him that we were on our way to the hospital. He was delighted to hear the news. As for me, I was simply glowing!

Junior is six months old now. I haven't had a decent night's sleep. My nipples are so sore. This little guy has an absolutely insatiable appetite. I never want to hear the word sex again. I'm constantly changing diapers and wiping up spit-up. I don't even have the energy to microwave those wonderful meals waiting in the freezer. It seems that whenever I finally find a few minutes to relax in a bath or call up a friend, Junior screeches at the top of his lungs. Other than doctor appointments, we haven't been in the car. We still haven't made it to the park.

The other day I told my husband that we should hire a nanny. I was going stir-crazy staying home with Junior. The house was a mess. I had my hands full just cleaning up the baby, never mind the rest of the house. Laundry was piled up everywhere. Food was rotting in the fridge. I often locked myself in our bedroom and just cried my heart out, and that didn't even drown out Junior's screams. My entire personality changed. I was agitated, starting smoking again, and had developed quite a temper.

When the doctor asked me if I felt sad, I laughed hysterically. Sad was not the word I would use. It was more like drowning in quicksand and never being able to get out. I had lost weight, never wore makeup anymore, and constantly grabbed clothes out of the laundry hamper. I couldn't have cared less how I looked. I didn't have the energy to go out.

My doctor smiled and said that I was experiencing post-partum depression. He patiently explained the condition to me and gave me a prescription. He told me to come back in two weeks and we'd take it from there. I felt a little better after that appointment. I had a condition that other women had too. He didn't treat me like a spoiled child who was just jealous of all the attention Junior got.

Junior is eleven months old now. I have gradually started to feel better since that first appointment five months ago. I'm actually looking forward to making Junior his first birthday party.

So if any of you have been going through what I have, maybe my story might help you to find the pot of gold at the end of the rainbow.

*****

I am never ever having another baby. I have never felt so miserable in my life. I walked around like a beached whale for months. I couldn't figure out where the weight came from because it seemed like I was always puking. My friends all said I'd feel much better when the baby was born.

Wrong! The kid is three months old and gets up a gazillion times every night. He gets a bottle. That way I get my husband to feed him too so I get a little bit of sleep. And the diapers! Yuck! I change him and five minutes later he needs to be changed again. And sometimes it leaks out onto his clothes! The sheets in his crib don't last a day either.

This kid has a set of lungs like you wouldn't believe! Half the time I can't figure out what he's crying about. I can't even throw him in the car and take him for rides because gas is so expensive these days. When he gets in the car he falls fast asleep. I wish he'd do that at home.

Pretty soon we're supposed to give him cereal and pureed fruit. The kid gets instant oatmeal and whatever fruit comes in a jar. I have friends who do their own fruit in a blender. I couldn't be bothered because you can buy it.

I can hardly wait until I go back to work. This kid is making me a nervous wreck. I cry a lot and scream at my husband a lot. This morning I just let the kid scream and stayed in bed with ear plugs and the covers drawn over my head to drown him out.

My house looks like a tornado hit it. There's no time to clean and I really don't have the energy anyways. It's getting to the point where I know all the take-out menus from memory. You just need to take a look around and you can see the empty containers everywhere. I don't even bother taking the garbage out anymore. That's way too much effort.

And I'm still wearing some of my maternity clothes. I haven't got my figure back yet, and at this rate I probably won't. If I had some decent clothes to wear I might even go back to work. Keep dreaming! I've just become a lazy slob.

I hate my life and I think I'll be stuck like this forever.

*****

Contributors' Stories Part 6: Eating Disorders

People say I'm anorexic. I think they're just jealous of my figure. They stuff their faces with burgers and fries. I don't. A salad is all I need. I'm five feet eight inches and I weigh a little under one hundred pounds. I don't see anything wrong with that. I wish people would just leave me alone.

My boyfriend broke up with me last week. He kept harping about how I never eat and he said he didn't want a skeleton for a girlfriend. What does he know? Big deal that he's the star quarterback on the senior football team. I think he's fat.

My mom wants me to go to a doctor for a checkup. She's worried because I haven't had a period for a while. I'm not. I don't miss them at all. So I don't see what her beef is.

My dad says I lie around and watch TV too much. He says I should go out for a walk and get some exercise. Or that I should come jogging with him in the morning. Last time I tried jogging with him I got totally winded before we even reached the trails. In the park. Then he got mad because I sat down on a bench and wanted to rest. He's a gym teacher and thinks that everyone should keep up with him.

Yesterday the guidance counselor pulled me out of history class. What nerve she has! She actually wanted to weigh me and have the home ec teacher talk to me about nutrition. Oh, that's just great! Someone else to meddle in my life.

Everyone says I frown a lot. They think I'm unhappy. Like there's anything to be happy about in my life. They say I'm starting to sound more cynical and that I piss everybody off.

But I bet none of them have older brothers who sneak into their rooms at night and get into bed with them. That's right. They've been doing it since I was thirteen. They told me if I ever let my parents or anyone else know about it, they'd really make my life miserable. Or they might just drown me in the lake.

At least they don't think I'm a skeleton. And if you put this in your book it better be anonymous.

*****

I have a friend who recently had staples put in her stomach. Just the idea of having someone carve out my insides and staple them together again makes me sick. I know I have weight to lose but I sure don't want to have that done.

My friend says it was worth all the pain. She's losing weight steadily and no longer has urges to eat an entire chocolate cake or a container of ice cream. Actually, she does look pretty good.

I've tried so many different diets and not one of them has helped. Sure, in the beginning I lost weight. But I was always hungry. And I could never stay on the diet.

Probably I just don't want to lose weight as badly as I want to eat. I think I'm addicted to food. I've heard the stories that I could become diabetic or that I'm likely to have a heart attack. But losing weight is just too hard. I enjoy my food too much. I'd rather go to a concert than be caught dead in a gym.

Now, here's the thing. I like to wear expensive clothes. I like designer labels. But I'm just getting too big to fit nice clothes anymore. I'm twenty-six and I weigh 283 lb. I'm just over five feet in height. Isn't that a pretty picture!

Men aren't attracted to big blobs like me. You think that would give me incentive to lose weight.

Got to go. My breadmaker just beeped. My morning snack is ready. A delicious loaf of banana nut bread. Now I need to decide if I want caramel sauce or whipped cream on it. Both might be nice.

*****

My daughter is seventeen now. For the last three years our lives have been a living hell. When she was fourteen, she was an outgoing and cheerful little girl. She had a lot of friends and was at the stage where she was becoming more and more interested in boys. She started to wear makeup to school and she was very fussy about the clothes she wore. All in all, she seemed like a perfectly normal teenager.

My husband and I had always wanted a large family. I have three sisters and he has two brothers and a sister. Unfortunately, I was only able to conceive and carry to term one baby. And that was our daughter Lyn. (That isn't her real name, but it's the name I'll use for writing this submission.)

Lyn was always a good eater from the time she was born, until the year she turned fourteen. Lyn had always been an average weight for her height and body build. But I started to notice that along with the makeup and designer clothes, she was starting to eat less and to lose weight. Lyn told me that she felt chubby, and just wanted to lose a few pounds. But those few pounds turned into more pounds. She began to look emaciated. Her clothes hung on her and she had started wearing long sleeved sweaters, even in the heat of the summer.

Lyn was never athletic. But suddenly she started jogging every morning before school. She drank SlimFast, reassuring me that this was all a part of her new fitness routine. I was dusting and vacuuming her bedroom one morning when I found some empty laxative containers in her garbage can. I confronted her with these when she came home from school. Her explanation was that she had been constipated.

I got a phone call from the school guidance counselor a few days later. The school was now concerned about her weight loss, and one of the other students had reported that Lyn vomited in the washroom after having lunch.

This was the beginning of the nightmare. We have taken Lyn to doctors, specialists, psychologists, psychiatrists, counselors; you name them, she's seen them. There is such an air of tension in our home all the time. My husband has lost all patience. He loves Lyn very much, but he says he can't sit around and watch her die. He told me last night that he has found an apartment nearby and that he is moving out.

Lyn merely shrugged her shoulders when I told her this morning that her father was leaving us. Her attitude is that it will be one less person to bug her about eating. Lyn's immune system has all but disappeared, and she spends a lot of time at home with colds and flu. She wraps herself up in blankets and lies on her bed watching tv or listening to cds. She hasn't attended school this semester. She just has no energy.

I am a nervous wreck. Her eighteenth birthday is approaching, and I will then lose whatever hold I have right now. I am watching my little girl starve to death, and I feel so helpless. I don't know where else to turn right now. Lyn has spent time in two different hospices, and the improvement was only temporary. I can't remember the last time she had a period. Her breasts are not developing normally. Her hair is falling out. Her teeth are rotting from vomiting so much. Lyn's joints ache and she wobbles when she walks. She refuses to be hospitalized or to seek any more medical attention. Lyn says she'd rather be dead than to live a life where she feels fat and ugly.

*****

Contributors' Stories Part 7: Obsessive Compulsive Disorder

I was diagnosed with obsessive compulsive disorder when I was in my twenties. I'm one of these people that repeatedly do things over and over to make sure that they are right. I can't control my behavior.

I can spend twenty minutes washing my hands before I sit down to dinner. I like my clothes folded a certain way so that there are no creases. I spend hours putting away laundry in my drawers and closets. And that is after they have gone through the wash cycle three times and the dry cycle three times.

In my kitchen pantry all my items are arranged alphabetically. I do not stack soups or other cans. I put dates on all these items and always check three times to make sure that they are rotated properly when I prepare a meal.

At school I was always the last one to complete assignments. Going to the fountain for a drink of water was a whole process in itself. The fountain had to be cleaned properly first before I'd take a drink. And then I had to wipe out down after I was finished. That would take half an hour.

When I go to the gym to use the machines, I carefully wash them down several times before I use them and then several times after. Meanwhile, people line up behind me because they want to use that machine and there aren't that many.

I'm very tired now. This is my fourth attempt at preparing a submission for the book. And I still have to fold it and put it in the envelope and then pass it on to the friend who gave it to me so that she can pass it along and it will hopefully get to you.

*****

This is tough. My wife used to tease me because I'd always go back into the house several times before we would go out. Each time I'd check to make sure the windows were all closed, I'd make sure the tv was off, the oven was off, the coffee maker was unplugged. You name it. I checked it. My wife used to grab my house keys after I'd checked everything out several times.

I would drive everyone at work crazy because I'd do the same things over and over before I left. I'd check to make sure that my tools were put away properly, my work clothes hung neatly in the closet, my work boots on the floor with the laces tied together. It's a good thing I didn't have to punch a clock or lock any doors.

There were other things too, but I don't want to write about them. They really drag me down.

One day at work, my boss asked me if I was nervous about anything, or if I was having any problems at home. He thought I should talk to a counselor. It was covered on my health plan anyways, so it wouldn't cost me anything.

I didn't really want to talk to a counselor, but my boss evaluates me on the job every year, and I figured if I wanted to keep my job, I should play along. Looking back on it now, my boss was a pretty good guy. The counselor referred me to a support group. I had no idea that there were other people out there like me. Some of them were doing even stranger things than I was.

It takes a lot of hard work on my part, and a lot of patience on my wife's, but things are looking better. I take pills everyday and never miss a support group. My wife comes to some of my counseling sessions too.

I think you should print my story. Other people like me might think that they're the only ones. And they aren't.

*****

I'm in my early twenties and I'm going bald. Not entirely. But there's big patches on my scalp with no hair anymore. You see, I let my hair grow long when I was in my teens. Then, when I'd get nervous, I'd chew on it and then tug on it. I'd pull it out by the roots. I don't do that so much anymore.

My eyes twitch a lot. I went to a doctor to get my eyes checked. Nothing wrong with the eyes. He said it was nerves.

I can't wear much jewelry. If I wear anything around my neck, I just twist it and twist it until the chain breaks. Sometimes my fingers bleed. But I can't stop.

The same thing happens if I wear a watch. I break the band from fiddling around with it so much.

My bedroom at home is immaculate. I vacuum my carpet and my mattress at least once a day. I shine the windows and mirrors constantly. I like to have things arranged just so on my desk and my vanity. I have my clothes arranged in my closet in alphabetical order by color. It gets kind of confusing when a shirt has more than one color. I move it back and forth and back and forth and it still doesn't look right.

My boyfriend says I'm getting really weird. He says I shouldn't be doing what I'm doing. He says I need a shrink. I think I need a new boyfriend.

*****

Contributors' Stories Part 8: Suicide

I was 16 when my brother died. My father is a doctor and my mother is a teacher. It was a real shock to come home from school one day and see my ten year old brother lying on the bathroom floor with blood everywhere. I can still see the pained expression on his face. It will haunt me forever. I started to cry and called 911 and called my father who was at work. It wasn't until the ambulance arrived that I realized my brother had used a knife to slit his wrists. My father came home just as they were putting my baby brother into a body bag. The police started asking all kinds of questions. My mother came home sometime during this time. When the police left I just cried and cried and cried. I thought it was all my fault, because I always used to call him a pest whenever he wanted to tag along with me and my friends. Maybe if I'd paid more attention to him. But we were 5 years apart in age and we didn't even go to the same schools. My father must have felt totally useless. After all, he was a doctor. My mother kept saying over and over that she should have noticed that something was wrong.

One of my father's colleagues was a psychiatrist. He was an enormous help to us all. He told us that depression kills. Outwardly, my brother showed all the signs of a normal kid his age. He didn't have many friends but he was an above average student.

But there was something very wrong and he hid it well, until he no longer could cope anymore. I think it's about time that more research was done about depression. It's a physical condition, just like diabetes or cancer. Some people are able to get the right help and with medication they can live a normal life.

I graduate from high school this spring. I always wanted to be a doctor like my father. But I don't want to be a surgeon anymore. I want to be a psychiatrist.

*****

My son committed suicide when he was sixteen. That was five years ago, but to me it seems like yesterday. My husband and I hadn't seen it coming. He was our only child. He was a first grandchild on both sides of the family. He was cherished and loved by everyone. His younger cousins all looked up to him and enjoyed spending time with him.

He was an honors student and was in the school band. He played hockey and baseball. He was well-liked at school and in the community. He was learning to drive.

The week before my husband found him hanging from a beam in the attic, his best friend had died in a car crash. My son left us a note before he hung himself. In his note he informed us that not only had he and Greg been best friends, they had also been lovers. He just couldn't go on without Greg in his life.

Everyone was shocked when this got out. Except for Greg's parents and his sister. Apparently Greg had confided in them several months before.

There are so many 'maybe' and 'what if' ideas that constantly whiz around in my head. My husband and I went for counseling together. That didn't help. We grew even more distant from each other. We had to cope in our own ways. Our divorce was amicable. We are now trying to move on with our lives.

*****

The first time I tried to kill myself I was thirteen years old. I hated school and couldn't stand being cooped up in a classroom in June writing exams when I could have been out riding around on my bike outside. I got up one morning, got dressed, had breakfast, and left the house. As I was riding my bike towards school, I thought that if I had

58

an accident then I wouldn't have to write the exam. Then I thought, I would never ever have to write another exam if I had a bad enough accident. I deliberately rode my bike off the bridge and into the water. Two men were out in a boat and saw me. They came to my rescue. I did get to miss that one exam. Other than a couple of bruises and swallowing some really gross river water, I was fine.

I got my driver's license when I was sixteen. Not that my Dad ever let me have the car very often. We always fought over that one. My older brother got the car whenever he wanted it. One night after everyone had gone to sleep, I snuck downstairs and into the garage. Yes! My brother had left the keys in the ignition. I lifted the garage door as quietly as I could and backed down the driveway with my headlights turned off. There was no need to close the garage door. I'd just have to open it again.

I was enjoying my drive, puffing away on a cigarette, when I saw flashing lights behind me. I slowed down so that the car could pass me. But, it turns out he didn't want to pass me. He just wanted me to pull over. No way was I doing that! My Dad would kill me if he knew I had the car out in the middle of the night. So I floored it. I started to lose control and I sideswiped a parked car. Then I thought I didn't want to stay in this world any longer. I drove head-on into the side of a brick building. That time I spent a while in the hospital.

My parents said I needed to go for counseling. That was a complete waste of time. I can just imagine the bullshit the counselor fed them. Actually, it was kind of fun playing games with the counselor.

I managed to graduate high school alive. In my first year at university, I overdosed on pills the night before my first exam. This time I wound up in a psychiatric ward at the hospital. You would not believe the freaks I met there! Actually, some of them were scary. One guy tried to hang himself and would up with damage to his brain. I decided I'd never try to hang myself.

I was given pills in the hospital. I tried to fake swallowing them, but I didn't get away with it. After a while, I started feeling better. I had both individual and group therapy on a regular basis. By the time I came out of the hospital, I was anxious to get back to school and try to live a normal life.

That was five years ago. I have one more year left before I graduate. My big decision now is what to study after I get my degree in science. I'm thinking about maybe going into a graduate program. I really like labs and I think I'd enjoy doing research. I'm glad that I'm still alive.

*****

I am a volunteer at our church. For five years now, I have helped to set up the receptions that follow a funeral service. As you can imagine, I have seen many families in their time of grief. But this one particular family stands out in my mind.

A man had passed away, leaving a wife in her early thirties with three young children all under the age of ten to raise by herself. The widow had no family in our community, although the deceased had quite a few relatives. I noticed that the woman and her children sat alone at a table, while all of the relatives sat together. But then I saw that the relatives were totally ignoring the widow and her children. Not only that, but you could see by their gestures and facial expressions that they were purposely avoiding any contact.

As the reception wound down, I noticed our minister talking with the young woman. His daughter joined them shortly after and proceeded to take the children out to the playground. It appeared that the distraught mother was pouring her heart out to our minister.

I was in the kitchen washing up the dishes and returning leftover food to the fridge when our minister walked through the door. He was clearly shaken and asked if we could all gather around the table as he had something to tell us.

It turns out that the deceased had for some years run a business locally. Leaner times arrived, and it was obvious that he had overextended himself. One day, while driving to work, he intentionally drove his car into a concrete barricade in a construction area. He wasn't wearing a seat belt either. The note he left his wife said that she and the children would be better off with him dead.

His relatives blamed the wife for her husband's suicide. They gossiped and decided that she must have made his life miserable. They wanted nothing to do with her. She intended to sell their house in order to pay off the debts, and then she wanted to take her children and return to the small town in Ontario where she had lived before she got married. She told the minister that she felt like a pariah. She felt that everyone in the neighborhood was staring at her and judging her, not just the relatives. Once word of the suicide got out, the children's playmates weren't allowed to come over anymore. Her husband had died tragically a week earlier, but his family's life in our community had died along with him. The funeral merely sealed their fate.

The widow and her children did move away. Not even the minister heard from her again. I often wonder how the family is doing. Did running away from their home really help? Surely the woman must have made a few friends here. I find it odd that absolutely no-one has ever heard from her again. I only hope that she did return to her hometown, and that she did find the peace and comfort there that was so desperately needed.

*****

Contributors' Stories Part 9: Loss and Grieving

I got very depressed when my auntie died. My mother had died giving birth to me so my auntie adopted me. She and my uncle wanted children, but couldn't have any of their own. My father disappeared right after my mother died. I'm 35, happily married and have a child of my own now. I have never tried to find my biological father.

My auntie died on Christmas Day last year. We had all gone to midnight mass together, and it was such a beautiful night.

The next morning my daughter was up bright and early to open her presents. My husband and I trudged down the stairs, half asleep. But I felt something was wrong. I couldn't smell the heavenly aroma of coffee coming from the kitchen. This was a ritual that my auntie had taken over when my uncle died several years ago.

I tapped lightly on her bedroom door. There was no response. I walked into her room and she appeared to be sleeping very peacefully. Too peacefully.

The following days were a blur. We had funeral arrangements to make, we had to phone relatives and friends and this was definitely not the way I thought we'd be spending our holidays.

Although we lived very close to my auntie, it was a Christmas tradition that we move in with her during the holiday until New Years Day. This year was no different, except that my dear sweet auntie was no longer with us.

My six year old daughter kept asking questions until I thought my head would explode. I breathed a sigh of relief when it was time for her to go back to school.

Then began the job of cleaning out my auntie's house, my childhood home, and preparing it for sale. There were several offers of help, but this was something I needed to do myself. I donated her clothing to the homeless shelter. I hadn't realized that she had lost so much weight over the last year. I kept her jewelry for my daughter. I saved some kitchen items that she had baked so many delicious cookies and cakes with. Thank goodness she wasn't one for knickknacks. I wrapped up the Christmas tree ornaments carefully.

After that I just became too overwhelmed. I let my husband dispose of the furniture and appliances and find a realtor.

When my auntie passed away I felt like my mother had died. I was now an orphan. I never wanted to go out anymore, even to the grocery store. Memories filled my head and I cried constantly. I couldn't sleep. I couldn't eat. I even let all my houseplants die. I had no energy to cook or to clean the house. I would just lie in bed and stare at the ceiling.

One day my husband suggested that we go out for a drive together while our daughter was at school. I didn't want to at first, but he can be very persuasive. I wasn't even upset when our ride was to a clinic to see a psychiatrist. I don't even remember what we talked about. But I do remember the pills he gave me.

I've been off these pills now for several weeks. I never bothered renewing the prescription or going back to see the doctor. My auntie used to say that "Time heals all wounds". And I guess this is just something I need to do myself in my own way.

*****

I'm a single mom raising three daughters. My husband died last summer. His motorcycle hit a semi-trailer on the highway. The RCMP said he went through a stop sign and that the accident was his fault. That is very difficult for me to accept.

He was always a very careful driver. He didn't speed, he didn't drink or use drugs, and his motorcycle was his pride and joy. I just don't understand how he could have run a stop sign.

The only witness who is still alive is the driver of the semi. He claims that he didn't see the motorcycle. All he felt was something crashing into his trailer and that caused him to lose control.

Why would my husband deliberately run a stop sign and enter a highway with a semi approaching at high speed? I just don't get it. He must have seen the truck. In the investigation the RCMP asked me if he was depressed or upset about anything. I honestly believe that he wasn't either. He was just out for a ride on a beautiful summer evening.

My little girls are so young and I'm sometimes still overwhelmed and don't know how to answer their questions. I tell them that their Daddy is in heaven and that he watches over all of us all the time. We have all had counseling, but their Daddy's death still remains a mystery to me.

Until I make some logical sense of what happened, I just can't get this out of my mind. I toss and turn at night. I have very little energy during the daytime. I have gained a lot of weight from just sitting around. I'm so sad all the time that I can't even cry anymore.

I still have all his clothes in the closet and his car still sits in the garage. My sister was over the other day and told me it was time to get rid of all his stuff. But I don't feel that I'm ready to do this yet. I probably should do what she says, but I just don't want to.

*****

I just lost my baby. It's the third miscarriage I've had in the last four years. I always make it through the first trimester but never the second. I felt those babies in my tummy. I knew I was growing something special and miraculous. Maybe we told people too soon. Maybe we should have waited to order furniture and decorate the bedroom. Maybe I shouldn't have shopped for blankets and clothes.

I just don't know anymore. I just feel like I have to accept the fact that I can't carry a baby to term. I feel so sad and lonely after every miscarriage. I feel so empty.

When I had the last miscarriage, they put me in a room with a woman who had just given birth. I wanted to feel that joy. I wanted people to look at me differently and be happy for a change. It just isn't fair!

I want to be a mom. I know I'd be a good mom. But I want my own child. And I want my child conceived in love. No test-tubes. No adoption. Just a normal pregnancy and a normal birth.

I ate properly, I exercised, and I don't smoke or drink. Why does this keep on happening? In the time I have miscarried three babies, my sister had a baby and my sister-in-law has a toddler and a newborn.

I just hate family gatherings and holidays. I cry silent tears at the sight of my new niece and nephews. But when I hold them, it feels awkward. I long to hold my own child in my arms.

I don't care if they spit up or get ear infections or have diarrhea. I just want a baby of my own to take care of.

My husband keeps trying to cheer me up and keeps hoping that I'll want to try again. What does he know? Has he ever felt another human being growing inside of him only to have it snatched away again suddenly? Does he have to suffer in silence because no-one wants to talk about it?

And my mother-in-law keeps repeating over and over that nobody on their side of the family ever had a miscarriage. That sure doesn't help either.

The other day my doctor mentioned that therapy might help. My husband laughed and said he wasn't going to pay for any 'quack' that couldn't do anything anyway.

I feel numb. I can't eat. I can't sleep. And I have no interest in anything going on around me anymore. My friends have given up calling me. I dropped out of my yoga class. I just don't know what to do anymore.

*****

My auntie came over one day. She told my mom she wrote you a story about being sad. She said her story would go in a book. I told her I can write a story. My hamster died. His name was Bucky. He was almost as old as me. I was real sad. Bucky was my best friend. He liked me. I liked him. My dad told me Bucky got old and then he died. I guess hamsters are like people. My grandpa died too. I was very sad. But now I'm all better. I'm not sad anymore. My grandpa is in heaven and Bucky can live with him. My dad told me we can buy a new pet. This time I want a bird. They are neat. And they sing. The cage can stay in my room like

Bucky did. I need to get a new name for my bird. My dad is going to work. He can mail my story to you. I can read it in your book.

*****

My wife died several years ago. We had been married for over thirty years. Together we had raised our children, enjoyed our grandchildren, and were still as much in love as the day we got engaged.

I was very lonely at first. I went to a grief support group at our church, and that is when I really started to heal. I began to attend church services regularly, and tentatively started to attend other church events too. Turning to religion really helped me. I always felt so at peace when in church.

But the comfort of the church was not all I found. As I became friendly with more and more members of the church, I then found a lovely woman whose husband had passed away a year before my wife. We began to spend more and more time together. My family all liked her, and her family felt the same way about me.

After what seemed like a whirlwind romance to everyone but the two of us, we eloped together. We were like two giddy teenagers when we came home. And we loved every minute of it!

We've been together now for almost three years. We attend church regularly and my wife teaches Sunday school. She even has me ballroom dancing now!

So for all of you who have lost a loved one, renew your faith in Jesus Christ, and I hope that you will be blessed as I have.

*****

Contributors' Stories Part 10: Manic Depressive

One day I received a phone call from my son's teacher. She was very concerned about his disruptive behavior in the classroom. He was becoming more aggressive and violent to the extent that she now found him a threat to herself and the other students. Quite frankly, I wasn't surprised. This past week especially, he seemed to be angry all the time. He seemed to fly into a violent rage if he didn't get what he wanted. He was exhibiting the role of a two year old rather than a sixteen year old.

There was no chance to speak to him that evening. He came storming through the door, threw his car keys on the table, and stomped off to his bedroom. He refused to join the rest of the family for dinner. His two older sisters were as puzzled as I was. My husband suggested that I " do something about it." I sighed and thought that I should contact the guidance counselor at his school.

The following morning, the girls left for their university classes, my husband went to work, and I drove down to the high school. The guidance counselor was a pleasant young man who wore the same dress code as the students consisting of jeans and t-shirts.

He provided me with a lot more detail that I wasn't exactly comfortable in hearing. My head was swimming on the way home. How could my son be so aggressive and violent at times and then seem to change instantly to a happy young man so excited about making the football team and going to parties? It just didn't make sense. I wondered if he was experimenting with drugs. The guidance counselor had suggested that I make an appointment for him with our family doctor. Perhaps there was a physical reason to explain this strange behavior. Oh please, don't let it be drugs!

Thankfully, the tests proved that he wasn't playing games with drugs. The only option now was to consult with a psychiatrist. And to persuade my son that he needed help. Believe it or not, the former was much more difficult than the latter.

After several months of waiting to see a professional and hours of psychological testing, a diagnosis was finally provided by a psychiatrist. I was astonished to hear her opinion. My son was bipolar! Unfortunately, this meant that he could not control his behavior on his own. He would probably be affected by this condition for the rest of his life.

The psychiatrist explained to us that our son was experiencing periods of extreme manic behavior and extreme depressive behavior. Treatment would include prescription medication and counseling. She told us not to expect immediate results. It would take a while before we would notice any definitive changes. At this point I didn't know whether to laugh or cry. I was relieved that he wasn't experimenting with drugs, drinking excessively or smoking pot. Our son was never going to be your typical teenager.

But this story does have a more positive twist to it. Our son is now eighteen and realizes that the pills and the psychiatrist will go hand in hand for some time to come. His behavior has improved somewhat, and he is even thinking about going to university now.

The real challenge will be when he moves out on his own and his family is no longer able to monitor him daily. Unlike his sisters, he wants to live near the campus in an apartment with his friends. We'll cross that bridge when we come to it.

*****

Mental illness seems to run in my family. Both of my parents have been on medication for depression ever since I was a kid living at home. I'm now in my thirties. My grandmothers on both sides of the family experienced dementia while they were in their late sixties.

Thinking about this makes me really feel down. I am afraid to have a serious relationship with a man, because that leads to marriage and marriage leads to children. I hate to think what kind of monsters I'd give birth to.

About ten years ago I was diagnosed as manic-depressive. I was relieved because my condition had a name. I knew it was different from the way my parents had been depressed. As long as they took their medication regularly they were fine. When they didn't there'd be a lot of yelling and fighting going on. And sulking in the bedroom. Once my dad even missed several weeks of work because he was so down.

I felt very different. There were days where I was so upbeat about life. I could multitask and enjoy everything. I'd laugh a lot, mostly too loud. I had all this energy and the sky was the limit. These were the good days.

The bad times would hit suddenly and without warning. If I had been enthusiastic about going to a concert, then all of a sudden I just wanted to stay home and sleep. My friends would get annoyed. It was my idea to go to the concert, I talked them into it, and then I refused to go.

It wasn't just concerts either. These black moods would just screw up my entire life. I didn't really need that haircut, and they wouldn't miss me at work today, and so on and so on. I was a regular Jeckyll and Hyde.

I can't remember how long I lived like this. Until one day one of my friends actually dragged me along with her when she went to see her shrink. I thought we were going for pedicures and was totally floored when she drove into the parking lot at the medical center.

Looking back on it now, it was probably a good thing. It took a while, but once I thought that therapy and drugs might help, I grew committed to the program. But it's hard work, and occasionally I really screw up.

I've had the same boyfriend now for over a year and we've decided to try living together. He is very supportive of me and I really enjoy being with him. We might even decide to get married someday. I'm still not sure about children.

*****

When my friend passed on an envelope from you requesting stories, I just had to write about my cousin. Thankfully his story has a happy ending.

I moved back to Toronto when I was in my forties. I hadn't been back since I was a teenager. I had kept in contact with one cousin. He had been married and divorced twice. He had two children with each wife, but he was estranged from all of them.

We had kept in touch by snail mail and then by email. His letters were always interesting but I always had the feeling that he had a tendency to exaggerate. He also talked about some pretty hair-brained schemes and I only hope that he had never followed up on them.

Now that I was back and we spent time together, I noticed some pretty alarming behaviors. He would call me up all excited about seeing a movie. We'd plan to meet later on in the week at the theatre. However I would often receive a phone call canceling our plans as he was too tired to go out or that he was feeling sick.

Sometimes I'd hear from him four or five times a week. Sometimes we'd connect about four or five times in a month. He had this annoying habit of not returning messages left on his voice-mail.

He had just started a new job when I moved back. By the time I'd been in Toronto for a year, I had given up on counting the number of jobs he had attempted. He just couldn't seem to hold on to a job. Actually, his whole life seemed rather chaotic to me. I never knew if plans I made with him would actually happen. Sometimes the weekends went smoothly and we did attend movies, concerts, parties, etc. But other times plans were cancelled at the last minute for no apparent reason. I had long suspected that the excuses of being too tired or feeling sick were not really valid.

My wife was a little more objective than I was. She was concerned that there was a definite mental health problem with my cousin. She pointed out how his moods seemed to swing from deliriously happy to overly depressed. She also mentioned that this condition seemed to be getting worse. At first I disagreed with her views. But as I spent more time with my cousin, things were becoming more obvious.

One of my coworkers had a brother who was a psychiatrist. I spoke to this doctor at length one day, describing some of the unusual behaviors and moods that I had noticed. He agreed to meet with my cousin.

Looking back on that day, I am glad that I arranged this session for my cousin. He has changed so much in the last couple of years. He attends regular therapy sessions, takes prescribed medications as directed, and his mental health has really improved. His days of bouncing from job to job are now over. He has a new woman in his life and they appear to have a great relationship. My wife and I see them quite often, and we always enjoy ourselves. Were it only that simple for others who are afflicted with a manic-depressive condition!

*****

Contributors' Stories Part 11: Schizophrenia

To my wife,

I don't know what is happening to me. I feel like I'm outside my body and looking down at my life. Some stranger has invaded my body. He is moody, unhappy, and violent at times. He shouts and swears at his children and doesn't want them around. He doesn't want to get out of bed in the morning. He has no appetite. He has taken a leave of absence from work.

The worst part is that I have no control of my life anymore. I keep telling you that the voices in my head are making me do things. You just don't believe me. The voices are all telling me to kill myself. I see myself speeding around some curve in the road in my Jaguar and careening over the edge. But I don't want anyone else to get hurt. I think about drowning myself in our pool. I think about sitting in my car that is running, with all the windows up and the garage door down. I think about slitting my wrists. I think about taking a whole bunch of pills and washing them down with a bottle of rye. I'm a lawyer. I have contacts. I can get a gun anytime and shoot myself in the head. I think about jumping off of bridges, balconies, and roofs. I think about hanging myself from a tree limb. I think about drinking a bottle of Draino or bleach.

The voices also tell me that I don't need you or the rest of the family or my friends anymore. That's why I can't even make love to you anymore. I don't want any physical contact with you anymore. I can't stand the sight of you. I don't know why you bother trying to help me. It just annoys me. I just want to be left alone. I don't want to read or watch movies. I don't want to play games with the kids or watch their soccer matches or dance recitals. I couldn't care less about their schoolwork. And I wish you'd just tell them to leave me alone!

And no, I don't want to see our friends or go to parties. And I definitely don't want to see my parents and my sisters, or your mother and your brothers. Have you any idea how hard it is just to go and see that psychiatrist that you drag me to once a week?

This story has taken me days to write and I don't feel any better for it. Like you said I would. I have nothing else to write.

From your crazy husband

*****

I live in a real run down area in the city. Lots of people living in the streets. They're always scrounging in garbage bins for food. They're so dirty. They smell really badly too, like they haven't had a shower or changed their clothes in months. Their hair looks scruffy.

There's this one guy who sits around on the sidewalk talking to himself all the time. He has a small wagon that he pulls around with all his things in it.

There's this other guy who always asks people for money. He says it's for coffee, but he stinks from alcohol.

There's a woman who shoplifts at a nearby drugstore. With all the security cameras in the store she gets caught a lot.

There's an open field nearby, and they sit around sniffing or drinking. They fight too. The police are always coming around. Sometimes they get hauled off to jail or the Sally Ann or the hospital.

There was this one guy who was always getting hauled off for exposing himself. He kept telling everyone that some angel lived in his body and that bodies are beautiful and shouldn't be hidden under clothes. I haven't seen him in a while though. I wonder if that angel is still with him.

This woman used to scream that there were rats crawling all over her body at night. I never seen any though. If it wasn't rats, it was bugs or birds pecking out her eyes. I never saw any of those either.

That's right. I used to be one of them. But not no more. There's this guy who's been coming around. He talks about God all the time. He helped me find some clothes that fit, got me a haircut, and took me to a shelter where I could shower and sleep. On Sundays he takes some of us out for breakfast. And he always preaches about God. He says he'll keep helping us if we stop sniffing and drinking. He says he'll show us how to help others too. Of course there is a catch. We need to work. The shelter needs some fixing up.

This guy is the one that gave me your envelope. He says he can tell I'm smarter than most. He thought I should tell you what life on the streets is like.

We aren't all bad people. Take me. I left home when I was in my last year of high school. I was never an honors kid, but I got by. My folks drank a lot, and one night my dad almost burnt the apartment down when he passed out on a chair with a lit cigarette in his mouth. Then my older sister started to be just like my mom. So I knew I couldn't stay there.

But after a couple of years on the streets, I was kind of glad when that preacher came around. I sure look a lot different today than I did a couple of months ago. But I do miss my friends from the field a lot.

*****

Author's Note

Tears came to my eyes several times when I read the stories that people had submitted. It was very difficult to choose which stories to include in **When Glad Becomes Sad.** This book has been quite an emotional undertaking and I feel that others are reaching out in search of support. It is my hope that you will take comfort in the words of others, and realize that you are not alone. My heart goes out to all of you, and my wish is that we all find peace and happiness in our lives.

Statistics From The Canadian Mental Health Association

It is often difficult to give exact statistics on the prevalence of depression in our society and the impact it has on individuals. Some generally accepted statistics are as follows:

It is estimated that 1 in 5 Canadians will be affected by a mental illness at some time in their life. More than 10% of the population aged 18 and over will have a depressive disorder. 20% of children and youth in Canada have a diagnosable psychiatric disorder. Almost 67% of homeless people have some form of mental illness.

Mental illness is the second leading cause of hospital use among those aged 20-44. It is also one of the most costly of all conditions in Canada. It is predicted that by the year 2020, depressive illnesses will become the second leading cause of disease burden worldwide, and the leading cause in developed countries such as Canada.

Treatments can be quite effective, but generally require lifetime use of medications. Only 43% of depressed adults seek care from a health professional. In Canada, 4000 people with major mental illnesses will die by suicide. More than 90% of people who take their lives have a diagnosable mental disorder.

Mental illness indirectly affects all Canadians at some time through a family member, friend or colleague. It affects people of all ages, educational and income levels, and cultures.

Suicide is one of the leading causes of death in both men and women from adolescence to middle age. The mortality rate due to suicide among men is four times the rate among women. Suicide amongst adolescents is rising.

Although depression can be treated effectively, there are too many people who are reluctant to seek help or admit to others that they are experiencing this condition and are receiving treatment. Yet the cost of mental illnesses in Canada for the healthcare system is well into the double digits of billions of dollars. This does not include the uninsured mental health services or the time taken off work by people suffering from depression. The latter is the fastest growing category causing losses in the economy of Canada.

Canada does not have sufficient resources to meet the needs of people who require these services, especially in the rural areas.

Medical Terminology

Agoraphobia occurs when a person avoids situations where a panic attack may be triggered.

Anorexia is a term used to describe an individual who experiences a loss of appetite that results in weight loss due to an unrealistic body image and low self-esteem.

Anxiety Disorder is characterized by a feeling of anxiety which affects behavior, thoughts, emotions and physical health.

Bipolar Disorder is also known as manic-depressive, periods of serious depression (lows) followed by markedly elevated or irritable moods (highs) not as a result of drug or alcohol usage. When people are manic social boundaries can deteriorate resulting in impulsive and reckless behavior that is uncharacteristic of them.

Bulimia is characterized by binge eating (when individuals consume large amounts of food) and vomiting.

Major Depression affects an individual's feelings, appetite, sleep pattern, concentration, memory, energy and ability to function over an extended period of time. Suicidal thoughts and behavior are common in depressive disorders.

Mood Disorder is a common term to describe individuals with a manic-depressive disorder or a bipolar disorder.

Obsessive Compulsive Disorder is an anxiety disorder where obsessive thoughts and/or compulsive behaviors are present to a degree which causes emotional or functional difficulties.

Panic Attack results from feelings of anxiety. It occurs without warning, is accompanied by sudden feelings of terror, may include chest pain, heart palpitations, shortness of breath, dizziness, feelings of unreality and fear of dying.

Phobia describes a fear of social situations or a specific phobia such as fear of heights.

Postpartum Depression occurs after a woman gives birth. It is characterized by despondency, tearfulness, feelings of inadequacy, irritability, mood swings and fatigue.

Post Traumatic Stress Disorder is also known as PTSD, a psychological event where serious harm occurred or a threatening or traumatic event was witnessed. Examples of these events are personal assaults, military combat or natural disasters.

Schizophrenia is a disorder characterized by hallucinations (otherwise commonly known as hearing voices) and delusions (belief system not based on reality). Other consequences are apathy, social isolation as well as relationship and occupational dysfunction.

Seasonal Affective Disorder is also known as SAD, when seasons of the year affect functioning of an individual and may cause periods of incapacitation. This is most common in the fall and winter when daylight hours are shorter.

Substance Abuse involves the use of drugs and/or alcohol to the extent that they cause chaotic relationships and/or occupational dysfunction.

Common Pharmaceutical Medications

Please note that the following are only some of the more common drugs on the market that are used to treat depression and anxiety.

Depression:
Effexor
Wellbutrin
Zoloft
Celexa
Prozac
Paxil

Anxiety:
Clonazepam
Lorazepam
Temazepam
Diazepam
Alaprazolam

All of the antidepressants are also used to treat anxiety.

References for Statistics

Unique News Winter 2007 from The Canadian Mental Health Association

Winnipeg Free Press article of January 12, 2008 quoting from The Mood Disorders Society Of Canada and The World Health Organization.

Recommended Reading

There are literally hundreds of books dealing with depression and anxiety that are available in bookstores, libraries and on the internet. Be sure to check out the books in department and discount stores. Other great places to find books are garage sales, flea markets, estate sales, auctions, and thrift stores. There are books available for people of all ages, including young children. Books can be found that are very technical and specific or very simple and general. For those of you who do not enjoy reading, you may choose to listen to audio recordings of books.

As mental health issues become more prominent in our society today, many magazines often feature interesting articles with valuable information. First person stories are becoming more common and are now more widely read than ever.

Other good sources of reading materials are medical professionals, spiritual leaders, educators, friends, and colleagues.

Additionally, in the Resources section that follows, a number of web sites are listed that contain very useful information. The agencies listed in this section will also assist you in finding appropriate reading material.

I sincerely hope *When Glad Becomes Sad* is a valuable addition to your library.

Resources

Anxiety Disorders Association of Manitoba
Phone 1-204-925-0600 Winnipeg
1-800-805-8855 (Toll-Free)
Web site www.adam.mb.ca

B.C. Partners for Mental Health and Addictions Information
Web site www.heretohelp.bc.ca

Bayridge Anxiety and Depression Center
Web site www.bayridgetreatmentcenter.com

Canadian Mental Health Association (National)
Web site www.cmha.ca

Canadian Mental Health Association (Manitoba Division)
Phone 1-204-953-2350
Web site www.manitoba.cmha.ca

Canadian Mental Health Association (Winnipeg)
Web site www.cmhawpg.ca

Depression and Bipolar Support Alliance
www.dbsalliance.org

Eating Disorders Self-Help Program
Phone 1-204-953-2358 (Winnipeg)

Health Canada
www.mentalhealthpromotion.com

Health Links
1-204-788-8200 (Winnipeg)
1-888-315-9257 (Toll Free)

Klinic Crisis Line
Phone 1-204-786-8686 (Winnipeg)
1-800-322-3019 (Toll Free)
Web site www.klinic.mb.ca

Manitoba Farm and Rural Stress Line
Phone 1-866-367-3276 (Toll Free)
Web site www.ruralstress.ca

Manitoba Schizophrenia Society Inc.
Phone 1-204-786-1616 (Winnipeg)
Web site www.mss.mb.ca

Manitoba Suicide Line
Phone 1-877-435-7170 (Toll Free)
Web site www.suicideline.ca

Mayo Clinic
Web site www.mayoclinic.com

Mental Health Education Resource Centre of Manitoba
Phone 1-204-953-2355 (Winnipeg)

Mood Disorders Association of Manitoba Inc.
Phone 1-204-786-0987 (Winnipeg)
Web site www.depression.mb.ca

Mount Carmel Clinic
Phone 1-204-582-2311 (Winnipeg)

National Eating Disorder Information Centre
www.nedic.ca

Obsessive Compulsive Disorder Centre Manitoba
Phone 1-204-942-3331 (Winnipeg)
www.ocdmanitoba.ca

Postpartum Support International
www.postpartum.net

Rainbow Resource Centre
Phone 1-204-284-5208 (Winnipeg)

SAMHSA Health Information Network
Web site www.samhsa.gov/shin

Seneca House
Phone 1-204-942-9276 (Winnipeg)

Sexual Assault Crisis Line
Phone 1-204-786-8631 (Winnipeg)
1-888-292-7565 (Toll Free)

Teen Touch Help-Line
Phone 1-204-783-1116 (Winnipeg)
1-800-563-8336 (Toll Free)

Winnipeg Regional Health Authority
www.wrha.mb.ca

Winnipeg Regional Health Authority
Mobile Crisis Services
1-204-940-1781 (Winnipeg)

In addition to the agencies listed above, please check the yellow pages in your local telephone directory for hospital and community health clinic information. Many religious institutions and health care centers also offer support groups and counseling.